in

Dr. Asha T £ 5/95

An Aid to the
Paediatric
MRCP Viva

D0413727

PRITHVI BOOK AGENCY

22 FEB 2000

FORT B'LORE-2 ☎ 6791960, 6703939

To our parents
Mavis and Norman Tinklin
Chandra and Ramesh Shetty
Joan and Jack Cade

An Aid to the Paediatric MRCP Viva

Alan Cade
MBChB MRCP (UK) DCH
Research Fellow in Paediatrics
Department of Paediatrics and Child Health
University of Leeds School of Medicine

Arun Shetty
BSc MBChB (Hons) MRCGP MRCP (UK)
Principal
Plains View Practice
Nottingham

Tracy S Tinklin
BM MRCP (UK)
Registrar in Paediatrics
Queen's Medical Centre
Nottingham

Foreword by
Professor Sir David Hull
BSc MB DObst RCOG FRCP DCH
Professor of Child Health
Queen's Medical Centre
Nottingham

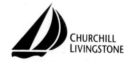

EDINBURGH HONG KONG LONDON MADRID MELBOURNE NEW YORK AND TOKYO 1995

CHURCHILL LIVINGSTONE
Medical Division of Pearson Professional Limited

Distributed in the United States of America by Churchill
Livingstone Inc., 650 Avenue of the Americas, New York,
N.Y. 10011, and by associated companies, branches and
representatives throughout the world.

© Pearson Professional Limited 1995

All rights reserved. No part of this publication may be
reproduced, stored in a retrieval system, or transmitted
in any form or by any means, electronic, mechanical,
photocopying, recording or otherwise, without either the
prior permission of the publishers (Churchill Livingstone,
Robert Stevenson House, 1–3 Baxter's Place, Leith Walk,
Edinburgh, EH1 3AF), or a licence permitting restricted
copying in the United Kingdom issued by
the Copyright Licensing Agency Ltd,
90 Tottenham Court Road, London, W1P 9HE.

First published 1995
    Reprinted 1996
    Reprinted 1997

ISBN 0-443-05246-8

British Library Cataloguing in Publication Data
A catalogue record for this book is available from the
British Library.

Library of Congress Cataloging in Publication Data
A catalog record for this book is available from the
Library of Congress.

The
publisher's
policy is to use
**paper manufactured
from sustainable forests**

Produced by Longman Singapore Publishers (Pte) Ltd.
Printed in Singapore

Foreword

The primary aim of this book is to help candidates to perform well in the final part of the MRCP examination, the viva. In this it succeeds admirably. The authors have asked candidates what they were asked, they have collected the questions and arranged them into some sort of order, and then they have prepared model answers. The text is peppered with helpful and often amusing asides about style, technique and the idiosyncrasies of examiners. It would be unfair to any candidate who has read this book for an examiner to look like a 'bored slump in his or her chair'. The candidate, he or she, might be asked what they find amusing!

The book can be read in bits, for example whilst awaiting the results of clinical investigations or a hoped for clinical improvement; it can be read for fun, just to see whether you would answer the question that way; and it can be read as a ready source of essential facts.

I was reassured by the breadth and balance of the questions as well as the answers. It has given me greater confidence in the value of the viva as part of the examination. I am a little reluctant to recommend that examiners should read it, lest they felt obliged to think of new questions to ask. However, it would be to their advantage for they would learn what sort of answers they might reasonably expect. Equally, I hesitate to suggest that it should be studied by the Examining Board, but I think it should, so that the viva is less of a 'turkey shoot', more an identification of the ill prepared!

What impressed me the most was that the exercise of preparing for the viva requires candidates to think through a number of issues which are not addressed in standard texts or review articles; what you would do, what you would say, how you would advise, how you would appraise. In preparing 'answers' the authors face the issues of the candidates' incomplete knowledge and understanding and the need to exercise judgement and selection. For these reasons I think this would be a valuable book for all members of a clinical service.

Some may take comfort in the thought that one of the authors did not pass the examination the first time. You would perhaps be right to conclude that this illustrates the limitations of the MRCP examination. No examination can be perfect, inevitably it will be unfair from time to time. The hope of the authors, which I share, is that this book will reduce the chances of the careers of paediatricians in training being unreasonably delayed by this artificial but essential hurdle.

1995   David Hull

Preface

The paediatric membership examination is a necessary, and for some, traumatic hurdle to overcome. There is no better tutor than that of hands on experience on the wards, in clinics and in casualty. For the clinical part of the membership great emphasis is placed upon the importance of the short cases and to a lesser extent, the long case. To this end, many hours are spent under the exam situation being 'grilled' on patients. Unfortunately, when the time comes 'for real', candidates can pass through the clinical cases but then fall at the last fence because of inadequate preparation for the viva.

It is true that the examiners can ask you absolutely anything from recent advances in gene therapy for cystic fibrosis to anatomy of the fetal circulation. However, provided you can answer in a structured, ordered and coherent manner, depth of subject knowledge is not required to pass.

The aim of this book is to provide straightforward, organised answers to the more 'popular' questions asked. It is *not* a book filled with factual knowledge and statistics, nor does it attempt to cover every possible topic in paediatrics. Instead, it can provide more digestible material to read in the small hours of the night, when children are even more unwilling to have their splenomegaly prodded, measured and diagnosed as a mesoblastic nephroma!

The very best of luck!

A.C.
A.S.
1995   T.T.

Acknowledgements

First and foremost, we must collectively pay special tribute to Dr Martin Hewitt (Consultant Paediatrician and Paediatric Oncologist) who painstakingly and ever-cheerfully read the entire manuscript. He is a fine teacher and without his guidance throughout, this book would not be on the bookshelves now. Not only have we enjoyed working with and learning from him on the wards but we have also had the task of writing this book made easier by a very generous man.

Special thanks also to our friend, Dr Tom Solomon (Research Fellow in Tropical Medicine) for writing the sections on PUO, HIV and malaria and also for his thoughts on the introduction.

Warm acknowledgement to Mavis Tinklin for her constant and enthusiastic assistance as well as moral support.

We are indebted to Dr Derek I Johnston (Consultant Paediatrician), Dr David Readett (Paediatric Oncologist), Mr Kevin Gibbin (Consultant ENT Surgeon), Dr Robert Walker (Community Paediatrician), Dr Jonathan H Shanks (Histopathologist) and Professor Elizabeth Newsome (Child Psychologist) for their guidance in their fields of expertise.

Thank you to Ros Waring for her secretarial skills.

Finally, special thanks to Franziska Kunick for her unique blend of warmth and encouragement and to all our colleagues where ever they may be... who make it all worthwhile.

Contents

Introduction

A paediatric MRCP candidate evolves from a very broad species but our research has revealed certain shared characteristics. He or she, though highly refined and intelligenced, is usually a very stressed animal, burdened by numerous evenings wiped-out by on-calls or their aftermath. There also appear to be two distinct subsets within the species. We have found a few individuals who hide themselves away with their objets d'art (a copy of *Forfar's* and a few piles of *Archives*), well in advance of the 2 months of torture. However, a second much larger group (. . . who are usually either fearful or suspicious of the first) seem to wake up one morning and discover that the turkey-shoot is only a couple of months away! This group then ponders the ensuing weeks in a daze of uncertainty, unsure of whether they should be spending their few remaining evenings attempting to drag an unsuspecting registrar or consultant around those all-to-infrequent 'hot-cases' or trying to chat-up the hospital librarian. It is at this point that they usually start digging away at the shelves in their local medical bookshop, frantically clearing away the mountains of colourful gems intended for their spoiled adult MRCP cousins, in an attempt to try and uncover those rare paediatric nutshells.

We have tried to write a user-friendly guide that will lend itself both to systematic absorption or to a frantic last-minute digestion and will therefore be of use to individuals from both of these subgroups. Our main aim is to provide the reader with a *system* which should maximise the marks obtained from the viva at whatever level of knowledge or experience he or she has attained. 'The viva system' is described in our opening section on viva principles and built upon in the following chapters.

Our second (and less important) aim is to present framework answers with some factual material to the commoner questions which arose from our survey of numerous examination candidates. We have divided these into sections so that the candidate may peruse a few topics in conjunction with his or her own formal preparation of that field.

Our answers are designed to provide an 'opening gambit' and it is important to realise that in the real viva, the flowing candidate will usually be interrupted at frequent intervals. Some of our responses are written in a progressive question–answer style in order to simulate this. (We have used abbreviations for the sake of brevity; generally they should be avoided in the examination.)

From our own recent experiences, the viva (after the short cases) is the second most daunting component of the membership examination. It is also, all too frequently, neglected under the misapprehension that you 'can't fail on the viva alone'. This is not the case and one of us (having passed the other sections) was floored by a viva on statistics and epidemiology. In addition, it is usual to be borderline in at least one of the other sections (often the short cases) and the viva is an ideal opportunity to gain valuable, even life-saving, extra marks.

We hope this guide will be of use in the unsettling and often unsteady journey to the membership (and beyond) and it is for this purpose that it is primarily designed. However, it should also be of value to medical students and DCH candidates.

Viva technique

Introduction

"... the viva was a terrifying ordeal. They can ask you anything so I didn't see any point in revising for it.

It is true that, potentially, you may find yourself having a talk about anything that is in *Forfar*'s or has ever been published in *Archives*. However, there are certain areas that are much more likely to crop up than others and we give a flavour of these in the main text of the book.

More importantly, we believe that good viva technique can be learnt (no matter how nervous or disorganised in thought you feel you are). In the viva, it is not just what you say but how you say it that counts. We have conducted numerous mock vivas in Nottingham and it is apparent that certain candidates with a relatively superficial depth of knowledge can viva infinitely better that others with a thorough reading, if armed with confidence and good technique.

We cannot stress enough that 3 or 4 hours spent in *mock vivas* (with any willing and motivated colleague) before the exam, practising what you glean from this book, will pay far more dividend than spending the equivalent time wading through obscure articles . . . (although important, most candidates over-estimate the required amount of journal experience). Make these as formal as possible, including having two slightly hawkish 'examiners', a desk, a knock on the door and a priming, "I hope you had a smooth journey to London". Try it! After a while they can be quite enjoyable experiences for candidate and 'examiner' alike.

The viva format

During the clinical section of the membership examination, you will encounter no less than six college examiners — two in the short cases, two in the long and two in the viva. The viva will last 20 minutes and will either be conducted in a quiet room or occasionally in a large hall. Though the latter is not ideal, most candidates usually say that you quickly become unaware of your surroundings.

One examiner will usually welcome you and may offer a handshake (do not offer yours first). You may be eased in with a social, "How was this morning?". Reply politely and avoid converting this into a long rambling chat. The examiners will then take 10 minutes each to bounce you around between different topics and test your mental agility. The other may well scribble away while you are in full flight. Do not be put off! This is normal.

The first question will often be on a broad topic to ease you in gently and to allow your tongue to warm up. Try and settle down and relax during this time.

The College seems to use the viva to test areas that cannot readily be assessed in other parts of the examination. These are:

1. Emergency paediatrics
2. A referral (from a GP or hospital colleague)
3. Social paediatrics, ethics, epidemiology and management
4. Basic sciences (relevant to clinical practice)
5. Recent advances and contentious issues (the journals!)
6. Hunt the diagnosis (what's in my mind?)

Above all, you must be solid and fluent when it comes to demonstrating your knowledge of emergency paediatrics.

You may also be asked a 'fun' question, often at the end of a viva. For example:

1. Tell me about an article which has changed your management.
2. What would you do with a research grant of £50 000?
3. Tell me about an important recent advance in the field of paediatrics.
4. How would you go about designing a neonatal unit?

The viva system

The examiner

There is no typical examiner. However, they are all practising paediatric consultants and are therefore generally a tamer breed than their adult cousins and should be amenable to a bit of charm. You will hear of 'hawks' and 'doves' and you should attempt to practise with colleagues from both species. You will probably find in reality that the examiner is in fact a myna bird and has the potential to resemble either species. Once practised, 'the system' can be used successfully to squeeze every last bit of 'doveishness' out of any hawk.

The candidate

On the day, you need to feel comfortable and confident and yet look smart and rather formal. Not easy!

Walk into the room confidently and smile when the examiners introduce themselves. Shake a pre-dried hand only when proffered. Speak with gentle confidence and avoid umms and errs. We make no apologies for reiterating the importance of mock vivas.

Sit straight! The examiner may well be in a bored slump in his or her chair. This is not an excuse to relax your attitude. Avoid attempts to simulate wild geese trying to take-off at the sight of a double-barrel . . . Keep flapping hands firmly under control on one's lap.

Aggressive body language will be noticed. The viva is about the examiners liking you and feeling happy to trust you with the charge of children. Allow yourself to see both sides of an argument whilst still gently expressing your own opinion.

When all is said and done, thank the examiners (they are there for your sake) and leave quietly without slamming the door.

All ears

You will probably still be reeling from the dreaded short cases. Thoughts of ". . . if only I'd remembered to examine for radio-femoral delay", keep trying to well-up in your mind. It is easy to lose half of what the examiner says in the heat of the moment.

Remember the battle is not lost until the examination is over. Put what is done firmly out of your mind and concentrate hard on your two new examiners and your current task.

Simple consultation principles apply. Always make eye contact with the examiner who is quizzing you.

All about confidence

From our discussions with membership examiners, we cannot stress enough how important a *confident* manner is for successful negotiation into the college. It is difficult to come across as firm and decisive but not arrogant or over-dogmatic, yet this is what is called for. Treat the viva as an intelligent discussion with a consultant colleague rather than a formal interrogation.

Another approach is to pretend that you are a paediatric SHO talking to a group of third-year medical students. Even if your teaching contains the occasional factual error, you will still come across as someone who is competent in the medical care of small children. Again, numerous practice sessions will help to fine tune your delivery style.

First impressions (your opening gambit)

There is more than a grain of truth in the adage 'it is the first 2 minutes that count'. What you are essentially trying to do during the whole of the clinical section is to prove that you are a confident and sensible doctor and would be a fitting colleague in the examiner's own department. If you come across this way during those initial 'getting to know you' moments, you are much more likely to be forgiven for later ruffles.

Answer approach

1. *Start with definitions*
Keep things simple for as long as possible. On the whole, the membership viva is not a test of small-print, detailed knowledge. It is more a test of how you handle this knowledge and confirmation that you have a solid understanding of the principles of paediatrics.

Where appropriate, start with well-accepted simple *definitions* (it may help to carry around a note book with definitions and opening gambits to the common paediatric topics). These sounds good and if you can switch to autopilot for a few seconds, you can use this time to plan the rest of your answer.

2.   *Show flare*

You need to sound like your responses stem from experience and 'the counsel of years', not merely from textbooks. Show flare and style! The examiner will have had to endure numerous nervous candidates already that day and he is likely to be preoccupied by what his hotel has on the menu for dinner that evening. The more life you can instill into your 20 minute allotted time, the more likely you are to eke precious marks from his thrifty nib.

"How would you manage a 4-year-old girl referred to your clinic with a history of urinary infections?"

Do not say:

"Well, eh, UTIs are quite an important problem in childhood and it is important to take a full history, carry out a thorough physical examination and then perform some investigations."

This sounds boring and, quite frankly, a medical student could trot it out. It also sounds like you are talking *at* the examiner. Try:

"This is a common problem and one which I have had to deal with on many occasions in clinic. I have come to realise that my first responsibility is to try and find out if these were genuine urinary infections as, if so, they can have far-reaching implications for a 4-year-old girl. Urinary infections in childhood may be of no real significance or they may indicate serious underlying disease where early discovery and intervention may prevent a lifetime of dealing with the dreadful spectre of chronic renal failure . . . ."

This sounds much more professional and should quickly convince the examiner that 'you know where he's coming from'. Note how the use of the first person "I would" makes for an altogether more authoritative and interested response. The second person produces a cold, depersonalised and somewhat boring answer.

3.   *Cast-off wide*

Start with an overview of the subject and only then feed the examiners some detail.

4.   *Structure your answers*

It is useful to *divide* up your response. This not only provides structure to your answer, making it easier for the examiner to tune into your thought processes, but it also makes you sound organised and in control.

"You are called to casualty to see a child who is fitting. What would your management be?"

"I would divide my management into first emergency procedures, including protecting the airway and controlling the fitting, and then subsequently determining the cause of the seizures. Thus, on arrival in casualty, I would . . ."

This division into emergency or early management followed by subsequent management can be used to make you sound polished in a variety of other situations. There are countless other ways of dividing up your answer and you should employ the technique or 'verbal headings' as much as possible. Scanty knowledge of a topic will sound much more voluminous and refined if what little there is, is classified!

5. Common things first
"Common things are common, rare things are rare." How often have you reeled this off to your medical students? Do not forget the principle when it comes to your own viva. When talking about erythema nodosum, make sure you talk about streptococcal and mycoplasmal infection, etc. before moving on to spout forth about the wonders of *Francisella tularensis!*

6. Steer the conversation
With practice and an agile sense of awareness of your *strengths* and *weaknesses*, you should be able to steer the examiner gently away from your uncharted waters towards those you are more familiar with. Once you have settled into a question and demonstrated a sensible start, throw out the odd bit of bait. Occasionally an examiner will bite, in which case you have the opportunity to really impress.

For example, imagine you have been asked about the principles of the management of chronic renal failure, a topic on which you are a little shaky. However, you have recently read a good review article on erythropoietin. Not at the outset, but after having presented a confident opening gambit and demonstrated a bit of experience and flare, why not drop in . .

"Anaemia in chronic renal failure is another important problem and its management has recently taken on a new lease of life since the introduction of genetically-engineered human erythropoietin."

The examiner, hopefully, will interrupt you with:

"Ah, erythropoietin . . . that's expensive stuff. Tell us something about it."

7. Avoid easy mistakes
Avoid the dreaded 'I think'. Why not try an exercise where you sit in the examiner's chair and question a nervous friend. You will quickly see how little confidence and style it instills when "I think" precedes every sentence.

If you are not certain that a point you are going to make is absolutely accepted in paediatric practice, why not prefix it with "I believe . .". This sounds more mature and comes across as opinion rather than uncertainty. (One of the functions of the viva is to show that you have formed sensible opinions in the areas where the jury is still out.) Also, why not try "In my experience . . ." It usually sounds great!

Do not open up a can of worms. It is crass stupidity to mention hypophosphatasia if you know nothing about it. Having said that, you are not expected to be perfect and not even the examiner knows everything. You will make mistakes and also have virgin territory uncovered. Being comfortable handling what you do not know is just as important as handling what you do. Here are some examples:

"My understanding of this rather difficult area is . . . . ."

"Of course, what I've said is nonsense. What I really mean is . . ."

8. *Have fun*

Above all, try and use all your experience and training to allow you to have the confidence to enjoy yourself! If you do, the examiners are likely to as well and your chances of being rewarded are multiplied.

Basic sciences and patho-physiology

1

Renal physiology

Q. Tell me about renal physiology.

This is obviously a huge subject and one that I can only briefly cover in the short time available.

Kidneys develop from metanephric mesoderm, identifiable from about 5 weeks' gestation, with urine being produced from around 20 weeks' gestation. The kidneys do not play a part in excretion of waste products in utero as urine produced is swallowed and 'recycled'. At birth the kidneys contain at least 1 million nephrons and do not increase in number through childhood, although infantile glomerular filtration rate (GFR) is much lower than adult GFR (25 ml/min/1.73 m² vs 150 ml/min/1.73 m²). Adult values are reached by around the end of the first year of life.

The kidney is involved in:

1. Electrolyte homeostasis
2. Acid–base balance
3. Hormone production — erythropoietin, renin, 1,25-dihydrocholecalciferol, prostaglandins
4. Excretion of end products of metabolism

25% of cardiac output flows to the kidneys. Filtration occurs at the glomerulus with passage of everything except blood cells and plasma proteins into the tubular system in normal health. Tubular reabsorption and secretion result in a much reduced volume of fluid produced as urine, containing only those products not required by the body. The basement membrane of the glomerulus allows particles of <8 nm in diameter through (equivalent to a molecular weight of 60 000) as a passive process. Control of GFR is dependent upon the capillary hydrostatic pressure, capillary permeability, renal blood flow and plasma albumin concentration.

The proximal tubule is the site of 70–75% of water and sodium reabsorption. The absorption of sodium is an active process; anions and water flow passively. Further sodium and water reabsorption occurs throughout the rest of the kidney tubule and collecting ducts but by different mechanisms.

The counter-current mechanism is employed to concentrate urine. Water is reabsorbed from the descending loop of Henle, thereby making tubular filtrate hypertonic by the time it reaches the medulla. The ascending loop is impermeable to water, but chloride is actively reabsorbed with sodium following passively. Urine entering the distal tubule is now hypotonic. Aldosterone produced in response to hyponatraemia by the adrenal cortex causes active reabsorption of sodium from the distal tubules and collecting ducts. This is a fine-tuning process as only about 10% of filtered sodium reaches the distal tubule. Aldosterone production is under the influence of renin secreted by the kidney juxta-glomerular apparatus in response to low blood pressure, hyponatreamia and hypovolaemia.

Anti-diuretic hormone secretion from the pituitary gland alters permeability of the collecting ducts to water and thereby alters tonicity of urine produced.

All filtered glucose should be reabsorbed in the normal kidney by an active process in the proximal tubule.

Urea is excreted by the kidney, associated with the counter-current mechanism.

Acid–base regulation involves bicarbonate absorption and H^+ secretion, the former taking place mainly in the proximal tubule and the latter in the distal tubule and collecting ducts. A fall in urine pH to 6 can be achieved by reabsorption of bicarbonate alone, but a further reduction requires H^+ secretion.

Erythropoietin is produced by peri-tubular cells of the renal cortex in response to hypoxia. 1,25-dihydrocholecalciferol is produced in the kidney by hydroxylation of 25-hydroxycholecalciferol. 1,25-DHCC is the active vitamin D metabolite and acts on:

1. The gut to regulate calcium and phosphate absorption
2. The kidney to regulate calcium and phosphate excretion
3. The bone to regulate calcium mobilisation and exchange with serum calcium

25-HCC hydroxylation is stimulated by parathyroid hormone release.

Prostaglandins produced by the kidney as a response to renal ischaemia are involved in renal blood flow regulation. They may have a role in modification of antidiuretic hormone action.

Haemoglobin and the oxygen dissociation curve

Q1. Tell me about haemoglobin.

Haemoglobin is a highly specialised and evolved molecule which increases the oxygen transporting capacity of a litre of blood from 5 to 250 ml. It also has a vital role in the transport of carbon dioxide and hydrogen ions.

The haemoglobin molecule is almost spherical and consists of four subunits, each consisting of a polypeptide chain (the globin) and a haem group. The polypeptide chains are of two types: α and β and there are two chains of each type. Adult haemoglobin (HbA) is therefore denoted $\alpha_2\beta_2$. A haem group (which gives haemoglobin its red colour) is associated with each globin chain and this consists of an organic part and an iron atom. The organic part, protoporphyrin, is made up of four pyrrole groups in the so-called tetrapyrrole ring. The iron atom binds to the four nitrogens in the centre of the tetrapyrrole ring and can take the ferrous +2 or ferric +3 form. Oxygen binds to the haem and this can only take place when the iron is in the ferrohaemoglobin +2 form. Each haem can bind one molecule of oxygen so one molecule of haemoglobin can transport four oxygen molecules. Ferrihaemoglobin is also known as methaemoglobin.

Haemoglobin is the classic example of a protein that exhibits *allosteric* properties. The binding of one molecule of oxygen enhances the binding of the next and this is therefore also known as co-operative binding. In other words, the affinity for the fourth oxygen molecule is far greater than for the first. This also works in reverse with liberation of the last oxygen occurring far more readily than liberation of the first. The co-operative binding of oxygen by haemoglobin enables it to deliver twice as much oxygen as it would if the sites were independent. The affinity of haemoglobin for oxygen is also influenced by other factors such as pH, CO_2 tension, 2–3 diphosphoglycerate (2, 3-DPG) and local temperature.

Q2. What do you know about the oxygen dissociation curve and how does what you've already told me influence its characteristics?

The saturation of haemoglobin with oxygen depends upon the tension of oxygen in the blood and the other factors I have already mentioned. A graph of the percentage of oxygen saturation of haemoglobin on the vertical axis and partial pressure of oxygen on the horizontal axis yields an S-shaped or *sigmoid* curve with relatively flat relationships at lower and higher tensions and a linear up-slope in the middle. This characteristic shape is critical for normal oxygen transport and is a direct result of the *allosteric* properties of the haemoglobin molecule.

The affinity of haemoglobin for oxygen is *decreased* by an increase in CO_2 tension, H^+ concentration (more acid pH), 2, 3-DPG concentration and temperature and this produces a right-shift in the curve. A right-shift will off-load oxygen from haemoglobin and this occurs in organs and tissues where oxygen is required. In actively metabolising tissues where there is a high demand for oxygen, H^+ and CO_2 are present in high concentrations since they are the end products of oxidative metabolism. 2, 3-DPG is formed from the metabolism of glucose in red blood cells and is present in human red cells at about the same molar concentration as haemoglobin. One molecule of 2, 3-DPG can be bound per haemoglobin molecule (held between the β-chains). No binding is possible when there is complete oxygenation of the haemoglobin molecule (i.e. in HbO_4, as in the normal arterial blood), but binding can take place in partially oxygenated or deoxygenated haemoglobin with the effect being to lower the affinity for oxygen binding by a factor of 26. Without 2, 3-DPG, the curve would remain sigmoidal but shifted over to the left. This would still mean that haemoglobin saturation in the lungs would approach 100%, but little of this oxygen would be liberated when the blood arrives in the tissues.

Q3. What do you know about fetal haemoglobin?

Fetal haemoglobin (HbF) contains two γ chains instead of the β chains in HbA and is therefore $\alpha_2\gamma_2$. HbF binds 2, 3-DPG less strongly than HbA and consequently has a *higher* oxygen affinity. This means that under physiological conditions, HbF is oxygenated at the expense of maternal HbA on the other side of the placental circulation. In the absence of 2, 3-DPG the oxygen affinities of the two haemoglobins would be reversed.

The liver and spleen are the main organs involved in erythropoiesis in early fetal life and they continue to manufacture blood cells until about 2 weeks after birth. The bone marrow is the most important site from about 6 months' gestation.

Bilirubin metabolism

Q. A knowledge of bilirubin metabolism is highly relevant to paediatrics. Tell me what you know about it.

Bilirubin is a tetrapyrrole compound formed when the ring structure of haem is broken open by microsomal haem oxygenase. It is produced mainly from the breakdown of mature erythrocytes which have a mean life span of 120 days. Red cells are removed extracellularly in the reticuloendothelial system (by macrophages in the spleen and bone marrow and by Kupffer cells in the liver). 15% of bilirubin comes from other sources of haem such as haemoglobin in defective immature erythrocytes, myoglobin, cytochromes and catalases. The iron and globin protein are separated from the haem and re-utilised.

The breakdown of haem yields carbon monoxide and biliverdin by the action of haem oxygenase. Biliverdin reductase is present in all tissues where haem breakdown occurs so biliverdin is almost instantaneously converted into bilirubin. (There is virtually no biliverdin detectable in plasma.) The bilirubin produced is unconjugated and therefore lipid-soluble and water-insoluble.

Bilirubin is then bound to albumin which renders it water-soluble and this complex is transported in the blood stream to the liver. Within the liver, the bilirubin dissociates from albumin and is taken up by the hepatic cell membrane and transported to the smooth endoplasmic reticulum (SER) by cytoplasmic carrier proteins. The process of conjugation then takes place where free bilirubin is bound to glucuronic acid by the action of the enzyme glucuronyl transferase (which is present within the SER). Each bilirubin molecule binds two glucuronic acid molecules. Bilirubin glucuronide is water-soluble and is actively transported against a concentration gradient into bile canaliculi and excreted into the intestine with the bile. A small amount of bilirubin glucuronide escapes from the liver which accounts for the low level of conjugated or 'direct' bilirubin which is normally detectable in serum (the normal value being 0–3.4 μmol/1).

In the terminal ileum, bacterial enzymes hydrolyse the conjugated molecule releasing free bilirubin which is then reduced to a group of products collectively known as stercobilinogen (or faecal urobilinogen). Most of the urobilinogen remains in the faeces where it is oxidised to the pigment stercobilin (this is normal faecal pigment). A small amount of urobilinogen is absorbed by the terminal ileum and transported back to the liver via the enterohepatic circulation; most of this is re-excreted back into the bile. A small amount of urobilinogen spills over into the general circulation and is excreted in the urine. This small amount of urobilinogen, which is normally present in urine, oxidises to the pigment urobilin on standing which may therefore darken the urine slightly.

If haemolysis is excessive, unconjugated bilirubin production increases and swamps the hepatic uptake capacity. Because unconjugated bilirubin is not water-soluble and therefore normally all protein-bound, it cannot enter the urine. Patients therefore do not have bilirubinuria and the urine is clear when it is passed, hence 'acholuric jaundice'. It may darken on standing due to formation of urobilin from the high levels of urobilinogen present.

Urinary urobilinogen excretion is very variable in normal subjects. Urinary urobilinogen is increased in: haemolytic diseases when faecal urobilinogen production is greatly increased resulting in the hepatic re-excretion capacity of absorbed urobilinogen being exceeded; and hepatocellular damage such as in hepatitis and cirrhosis when hepatic urobilinogen excretion is impaired. A negative urinary urobilinogen has a high sensitivity and specificity with obstructive jaundice. In infective hepatitis, urinary urobilinogen excretion shows a predictable pattern in relation to the course of the disease. In the early stages, urinary excretion is increased indicating hepatocellular dysfunction (which produces impairment of urobilinogen re-excretion into the biliary tract). Later on, urobilinogen disappears from the urine indicating the cholestatic phase.

Plasma-conjugated bilirubin is increased in intra- or extrahepatic cholestasis when there is impaired hepatic excretion of conjugated bilirubin, resulting in increased over-spill into the blood. It is also increased in hepatitis. Conjugated bilirubin, being water-soluble, readily passes into the urine and 'bilirubinuria' can easily be detected by stick tests before plasma bilirubin begins to rise. Since bilirubin is a pigment, when present in significant amounts it darkens the urine, hence 'choluric jaundice'. In cholestasis, conjugated bilirubin excretion is reduced which results in decreased faecal stercobilin and hence pale stools.

Tips

- This is a classic example of a 'basic sciences' question which is becoming increasingly popular. The topics chosen will usually be those that have some direct *clinical* relevance to paediatrics (as is the case here).

- Once the examiners have assessed your competence in basic science, they will often lead you into case scenarios so that they can test your ability to explain findings from 'first-principles' (i.e. the pathophysiology).

Fetal circulation

Q. Tell me about the fetal circulation and the changes that occur around the time of birth.

In utero the fetus receives oxygenated blood from the placenta via the left umbilical vein. This blood mixes with deoxygenated blood from the baby's own portal blood to enter the inferior vena cava. Here further mixing occurs with deoxygenated blood from the baby's legs and lower trunk. Blood passes from the right atrium through the foramen ovale to the left atrium and then out through the left ventricle, having mixed with the small amount of blood returning from the fetal lungs via the pulmonary veins. This blood from the left ventricle is highly oxygenated and primarily supplies oxygen to the head and neck.

Blood returning from the head and neck via the superior vena cava again enters the right atrium but because of the haemodynamics, this blood mixes very little with the more oxygenated blood that supplies the head and neck. Instead, this blood passes through the tricuspid valve into the right ventricle and is then shunted through the ductus arteriosus to join the descending aorta. Hence, blood to the lower limbs is less well oxygenated than that to the upper limbs, head and neck.

The transition from fetal 'life' to independent existence is a process fraught with potential danger. In utero the fetus is completely dependent on a functioning placenta. Once the placenta ceases to function adequately, the fetus must ready itself for extrauterine life. As a part of these changes the circulatory system undergoes dramatic transformations. On taking the first breath, the pulmonary vascular resistance drops significantly and the blood supply from the placenta is interrupted. These two separate processes result in closure of the *foramen ovale* and constriction and eventual closure of the *ductus arteriosus*. It is thought that local 'hyperoxia' as a result of reversed flow of aortic blood into the ductus arteriosus is the initiating factor for ductal constriction. The closure of the foramen ovale is simply a result of a rise in left atrial pressure and fall in right atrial pressure, causing the septum primum to rest against the septum secundum.

Calcium metabolism

Q1. Tell me something about calcium.

Calcium is one of the body's essential minerals and must be accumulated by the growing child. 99% of the total body calcium is present in *bone*. However, calcium also has vital roles in cardiac and neuromuscular excitability, endocrine function, blood coagulation and enzymatic reactions. The remaining 1% of the total body calcium which is present in the various body fluids must therefore be closely regulated.

Circulating plasma calcium exists in two main forms. Only 50% of the total measured plasma calcium is freely ionised but it is this fraction that is biologically active and under homeostatic control. This is in free exchange with protein (mostly albumin)-bound calcium which accounts for about 40% of the total and the concentration of this fraction is determined both by albumin-binding site and calcium availability. The small remainder is complexed to phosphate and other anions. The normal total plasma calcium concentration is 2.20–2.65 mmol/1 and unlike phosphate concentration, this is not age related. Various calculations have been devised to 'correct' total calcium concentration for abnormal albumin levels and a commonly used formula is to add 0.02 mmol/1 for every 1 g/1 that the albumin is below the normal level of 40 g/1. Similarly, in situations where the albumin is high, 0.02 mmol/1 is subtracted from the total plasma calcium for every 1 g/1 above 48 g/1. However, it must be remembered that it is the ionised calcium concentration which really concerns us and direct measurement of free calcium may be required with significant disturbances of acid–base balance. This is because hydrogen ions compete with calcium for albumin binding and therefore acidosis depresses calcium ionisation and vice versa in alkalosis.

Calcium homeostasis is controlled by two interacting mechanisms, namely the parathyroid gland releasing parathyroid hormone and by 1,25-dihydroxycholecalciferol from vitamin D. They act at three sites — bone, intestine and kidney, to increase plasma calcium.

Q2. What do you know about the role of the parathyroid gland in calcium regulation?

The most important factor in controlling the level of circulating free ionised calcium to within a very narrow range is parathyroid hormone (PTH). This hormone is secreted by the parathyroid gland in response to a fall in free calcium concentration and, like 1,25-dihydroxycholecalciferol, raises free calcium levels. PTH does this by two direct actions on calcium metabolism.

1. It causes stimulation of osteoclasts, therefore increasing the level of osteolysis and thus the release of calcium and phosphate from bone. (In fact, it is thought that osteoblasts possess receptors for PTH which mediate release of an osteoclast-promoting factor).
2. It acts on distal renal tubular cells to promote calcium reabsorption, hence increasing plasma concentration.

However, it reduces the reabsorption of phosphate thus tending to lower plasma levels; this is opposite to its effect on bone phosphate. This phosphaturic effect of PTH is not only physiologically important but an important action to bear in mind when it comes to understanding the pathophysiology of disorders of calcium metabolism.

PTH has a third indirect pro-calcium effect by stimulating renal synthesis of 1, 25-dihydroxycholecalciferol.

Q3. You mentioned 1, 25-dihydroxycholecalciferol. What do you know about vitamin D and its metabolites?

Vitamin D refers to cholecalciferol (vitamin D_3) which is synthesised in the epidermis by the action of ultraviolet light and ergocalciferol (vitamin D_2), which is plant-derived. As well as the endogenously-derived vitamin D_3, animal and plant foods are important sources of vitamin D_3 and D_2, respectively. Both of these are steroid-related, fat-soluble vitamins which are derived from cholesterol and, along with PTH, have a vital role in calcium metabolism.

They are transported in plasma bound to specific carrier proteins and are inactive until metabolised. The activation of vitamin D requires two hydroxylations, the first at the 25-position in the liver and the second at the 1-position in the kidney. This yields 1, 25-dihydroxycholecalciferol (1, 25-DHCC) which is the active form. Thus, this is one of the endocrine functions of the kidney with 1, 25-DHCC being the hormone.

1, 25-DHCC acts on intestinal cells to promote calcium absorption and on the kidney to increase calcium reabsorption. It also acts on bone (probably mediated by PTH), to mobilize calcium. In short-term homeostasis, the bone effects of PTH and 1, 25-DHCC are more important. The absorption from intestinal and renal tubular lumina is vital in the longer-term prevention of hypocalcaemia.

Q4. Do you know anything about 24, 25-dihydroxycholecalciferol?

Yes. Some of the 25-hydroxycholecalciferol arriving at the kidney undergoes hydroxylation at the 24- instead of the 1-position yielding 24, 25-dihydroxycholecalciferol. This has minimal activity compared to 1, 25-DHCC. As I alluded to earlier, PTH has an indirect pro-calcium effect on the kidney (as well as its direct one) by increasing the proportion of 1, 25-DHCC relative to 24, 25-DHCC produced.

Q5. You said that there are two main regulating mechanisms for calcium. Tell me something about calcitonin.

Calcitonin is a hormone which is secreted by the parafollicular C cells of the thyroid gland in response to high plasma calcium. The effects of calcitonin are opposite to those of PTH. It inhibits bone resorption and has calciuric and phosphaturic activity.

However, its physiological importance as a hypocalcaemic hormone in the older child and adult remains uncertain but is probably minor. Neither thyroidectomy nor calcitonin hypersecretion from a medullary thyroid carcinoma affect plasma calcium levels. It may be, however, that it has greater importance in the fetus and infant where calcitonin as well as 1, 25-DHCC levels are high. Calcitonin may have a physiological role here in preventing excess bone resorption and hence allowing the 1, 25-DHCC to promote intestinal calcium absorption.

Q6. What do you know about phosphate?

Phosphate (PO_3) is an essential part of most biochemical systems, including nucleic acids. About 80% of all body phosphorus resides in bone. Phosphate metabolism is very closely linked to calcium at a variety of levels, including their mutual bonding in plasma and in bone and their combined regulation by PTH and 1,25-DHCC. Unlike calcium, plasma inorganic phosphate concentration is age related in childhood, declining from high levels in infancy.

Q7. Tell me something about the interpretation of abnormal calcium or phosphate values.

Bearing in mind that calcium homeostasis is achieved at the level of the free ion and with a knowledge of the actions of the controlling hormones, PTH and 1, 25-DHCC, it is usually possible to unravel most of the derangements. In particular, I have found that the phosphaturic affect of PTH is one of the most important actions to grasp when attempting to interpret abnormal calcium or phosphate results. A low ionised calcium, unless due to hypoparathyroidism, stimulates the production of PTH and hence causes phosphaturia. The phosphaturic effect is greater than PTH's action on bone in mobilising phosphate and hence plasma phosphate levels will be low or low–normal.

As a rule of thumb therefore calcium and phosphate levels vary in the same direction unless the cause of the abnormality is either a disturbance of parathyroid function or renal failure (where the phosphaturic effect is reduced).

Cyanosis

Q1. Tell me about cyanosis.

Cyanosis is a clinical sign which means blue or purple discoloration of the skin or mucous membranes due to excessive deoxygenated haemoglobin in the blood perfusing the area concerned. In practice, at least 5 g/dl of deoxyhaemoglobin must be present for the colour to be observed.

Cyanosis is divided into *peripheral* and *central.* Peripheral cyanosis is caused by local vasoconstriction, usually due to a cold environment or shock, and occurs when any extremity is affected, but the tongue or buccal mucosa remain pink. The tongue and lips are resistant to the conditions liable to produce peripheral cyanosis as well as the sites closest to the aorta where arterial blood can be readily observed. If the tongue and buccal mucosa do show blue/purple discoloration, central cyanosis is present which may be due to either pulmonary or cardiac disease.

It is important to appreciate the difference between *cyanosis* and *hypoxia*, although the two are closely related. Cyanosis is purely a clinical sign. Hypoxia suggests inadequate oxygen supply to the cells for normal function. In an otherwise normal child, a low oxygen tension in arterial blood implies hypoxia and will lead to enough deoxyhaemoglobin to cause cyanosis. However, in severe anaemia, serious tissue hypoxia may be present without enough deoxyhaemoglobin (i.e. 5 g/dl) to produce cyanosis. Conversely, a polycythaemic child may be cyanosed, though not hypoxic.

Q2. What are the causes of central cyanosis?

As I have discussed, central cyanosis may be *respiratory* or *cardiac* in origin. I normally divide the respiratory causes into:

1. Pump problems
2. Exchange-surface problems
3. Airway problems

Pump problems are any cause of inadequate ventilatory activity. At the 'top end', these are depression of the respiratory centre from drugs, raised intracranial pressure or space occupation, cerebral trauma, intracranial sepsis, primary cerebral disease, etc. Diseases at the 'bottom end' include chest-wall abnormalities, diaphragmatic hernia, pneumothorax, etc. In between there may be neuropathy or muscle disease.

Airway problems include foreign body, large tonsils or adenoids, stenosis from croup, epiglottitis, pus, tumours and congenital causes, asthma and bronchiolitis.

Exchange-surface problems include pulmonary oedema, pneumonia, respiratory distress syndrome, cystic fibrosis, bronchiectasis and pulmonary fibrosis.

In other words, the pathophysiology of the respiratory causes of cyanosis is related either to a generalised reduction in ventilation (pump problems and major airway problems) or an imbalance between ventilation and perfusion within the lungs.

Most of the diseases encountered in paediatric cardiology have the potential to cause cyanosis at some stage in their natural history. The pathophysiology of cardiac central cyanosis is related to either a right-to-left shunt or cardiac failure. The latter cause by its nature occupies no-mans-ground between respiratory and cardiac causes.

I would divide the shunt causes as those that present with early cyanosis and those that may cause cyanosis later on. The early cyanosis group includes transposition of the great vessels and defects associated with reduced pulmonary blood flow (e.g. pulmonary atresia, tricuspid atresia and severe tetralogy of Fallot). Such infants usually have ductus-arteriosus-dependant pulmonary blood flow and inhibition of duct closure with an infusion of prostaglandin El or E2 may be required to stabilise the baby's condition whilst surgery is arranged.

The late cyanosis group is related to pulmonary hyperperfusion leading to pulmonary hypertension from chronic left-to-right shunting. This eventually leads to shunt reversal causing central cyanosis and digital clubbing (Eisenmenger syndrome). This group therefore includes VSD, ASD, PDA, pulmonary stenosis (with a patent foramen ovale) and atrioventricular canal defects.

Central cyanosis from heart failure may be related to coarctation of the aorta, aortic stenosis or hypoplastic left heart. It may also arise from any of the other congenital heart lesions if they are severe enough.

Q3. I'll stop you there. Briefly tell me how you would investigate a neonate with central cyanosis.

A knowledge of the above causes together with the child's obstetric and neonatal history and examination findings would guide my investigation plan.

Initial investigations would usually include a FBC, arterial blood gases and oximetry, a CXR, an ECG and an echocardiogram. I would also consider investigations related to sepsis, including blood cultures, U&E, blood glucose, urine culture and possibly a lumbar puncture.

In some situations, repeating the blood gases whilst administering 100% inhaled oxygen may help to identify the cause. Generally speaking, there will be no improvement in arterial PO_2 in the case of congenital cyanotic heart disease with right-to-left shunting. Central cyanosis due to primary lung disease or congenital heart disease with heart failure will show a response to the increased inspired PO_2. The test should be performed with caution in babies with suspected congenital heart disease as there may be reliance on patency of the ductus arteriosus, which will tend to close if the oxygen tension is increased. Facilities for prostaglandin infusion should be immediately available for reversing closure.

Q4. What do you know about methaemoglobinaemia?

Methaemoglobin occurs when the iron in the haem fraction of haemoglobin is oxidised to Fe^{3+}. This is 'functionally dead' haemoglobin (only reduced haem Fe^{2+} is functionally active) and various mechanisms are present within red cells to maintain the reduced form. Methaemoglobin is dark blue and may mimic cyanosis as well as reducing effective oxygen transport. Congenital methaemoglobinaemia is caused by absence of the enzyme metHb reductase. In addition, in susceptible individuals, various drugs and chemicals may cause methaemoglobinaemia, including sulphonamides, nitrates (e.g. in well-water), aniline and nitrobenzene.

Tips

- Another rather technical question which may 'separate the men from the boys'. Examiners seem to be keen on topics which span from physiology through pathophysiology to clinical medicine.

- As far as possible, keep things logical and simple and do not mention conditions which you know nothing about. Start with simple definitions and principles. They make you sound sensible and occupy time which may otherwise be spent discussing advances in the management of total anomalous pulmonary venous drainage!

Opsonisation

Q. What do you understand by the term opsonisation?

Opsonisation is the process whereby macrophage phagocytosis of antigens, particularly micro-organisms, is facilitated by their being coated either by complement or specific antibody. Immunologists talk about antigens being 'made tasty' to macrophages.

This function of complement is said to be one of the most powerful humoral defence systems and is largely mediated by C3b (the active component of C3), which has the ability to coat antigens. C3b acts as a powerful opsonin by binding to specific C3b receptors on macrophages.

There are reports of conditions where defects of opsonisation may occur in the absence of any of the antibody or complement deficiency states. An example of this is Leiner's disease which is recurrent infections in association with extensive dermatitis, diarrhoea and failure to thrive. The serum of these patients shows defective opsonisation in in-vitro studies (Jacobs & Miller 1972). To lend weight to this finding, fresh plasma infusions were found to improve the clinical condition.

Tips

■ A somewhat obscure topic, particularly from a clinical point of view, but one which appears to have been an increasingly popular discussion point in recent vivas.

■ It is likely that for most examiners, you merely need to demonstrate that you know what terms mean and have some understanding of their possible clinical relevance.

REFERENCE

Jacobs J C, Miller M E 1972. Fatal familial Leiner's disease: a deficiency of the opsonic activity of serum complement. Pediatrics 49: 225–232.

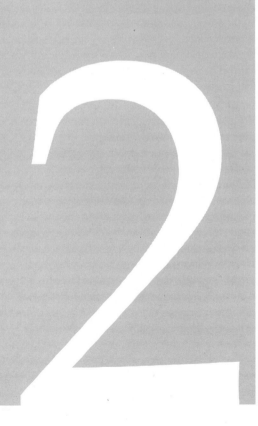

Emergency
paediatrics

2

Acute dyspnoea

Q. I want you to imagine you are the duty Paediatric registrar. Your junior SHO calls you at 2 am and says there is an unwell, very breathless, 14-year-old girl in casualty. Tell me how you would proceed.

The fact this girl is unwell concerns me and I would first ask the SHO to decide whether we need to crash call an anaesthetist. If this is not required, I would ask him to exclude a tension pneumothorax and organise blood gases, a BM stix and to put her on an oximeter whilst I am en route. I would also confirm that he has put her on high-flow (6 1/min) oxygen by mask. It would seem likely that she does not have obvious features of acute asthma (which would normally be the most likely cause of this scenario) as she has been described as 'breathless' rather than presenting with 'acute asthma'. However, I would confirm that, if she did, she had received nebulised bronchodilators. I would then go immediately to casualty.

On my way, I would run through in my mind the possible causes of her presentation. The *respiratory* causes are:

— acute asthma (this being the commonest cause)
— pneumothorax, including tension pneumothorax
— pulmonary embolism (PE)
— inhalation of foreign body
— severe pneumonia

Cardiac causes are less likely but include:

— cardiac failure due to an arrhythmia (the most likely being SVT)
— (outside possibility) cardiomyopathy (e.g. glue sniffers)
— high output failure from severe anaemia

Metabolic causes include:

— diabetic ketoacidosis
— salicylate poisoning
— uraemia.

Finally, a diagnosis largely of exclusion is *hysterical overbreathing* (hyperventilation).

When I arrive, I would first quickly ascertain whether she needs any acute life-saving procedures and, if necessary, administer *resuscitation* as per the European Resuscitation Council Guidelines. I would then specifically look for signs of a *tension pneumothorax* (hyperinflation, diminished expansion, hyperresonance and decreased breath sounds on the affected side of the chest with shift of the mediastinum — as judged by the position of the trachea and apex beat— towards the normal side). If this is the case, the acute life-threatening complication is loss of cardiac output due to embarrassment of venous return to the heart due to the mediastinal shift. I would therefore immediately insert a large intravenous cannula into the affected side of the chest. This will allow the mediastinum to centralise, allowing time for a chest X-ray and a chest drain.

If she is stable I would try to obtain some *history* from anyone accompanying her or the ambulance crew. She may be able to give me short answers and I would ask specifically about whether the breathlessness came on suddenly (asthma, pneumothorax, PE) or whether she had felt generally unwell recently (pneumonia, ketoacidosis), had any associated chest pain or palpitations, had any history of asthma, heart disease or diabetes, and whether she was on the pill (PE), had taken an overdose (salicylates) or had abused any substances.

I would then *examine* her, checking in particular her airway, breathing pattern, chest and pulse and look for signs of acute asthma (which should already be obvious), inhalation, pneumonia, PE (sinus tachycardia — unhelpful in this setting, possibly a pleural rub or signs of a DVT), endocarditis, heart failure and anaemia. I would also check for ketones on her breath and ascertain the results of her BM and urinalysis (for ketonuria).

I would then check her FBC, U&Es, ESR and blood cultures (if indicated), blood glucose, poisons screen, blood gases and chest X-ray (pneumonia, pneumothorax, air trapping if inhalation of foreign body). If indicated, I would arrange for an ECG to look for arrhythmias or features of a PE.

Careful analysis of her *blood gases* should help further to unravel the problem. If she is simply hyperventilating, I would expect a high–normal PO_2 with a low PCO_2 and possibly a respiratory alkalosis. If she has a metabolic acidosis this would also account for the dyspnoea and I would proceed by calculating her anion gap ((sodium + potassium) – (bicarbonate + chloride)). This should normally be about 12 mmol/1 (range 10–15). If high, this would point to ketoacidosis, salicylate intoxication or uraemia. A normal anion gap would be in keeping with an unusual diagnosis such as renal tubular acidosis.

By now, I think I would have obtained sufficient clues towards most organic problems and be able to manage her accordingly. If these are absent, I would consider the possibility of hysterical hyperventilation.

An unconscious child

Q. You are called to see a 13-year-old unconscious child in casualty. Run through your initial management of this problem.

On arrival in casualty I would perform any life-saving manoeuvres that are necessary, going through the ABC of resuscitation. Whilst doing this I would ask the attending nurse to carry out a thumb-prick capillary blood sugar and blood pressure measurement and to place the child on a cardiac monitor and a saturation monitor. If the child is in extremis or in need of immediate intubation and ventilation, I would seek the assistance of my paediatric anaesthetic colleague. Hopefully, there would be a relative or friend present or at least a member of the ambulance crew who may be able to shed a little more light on the situation; otherwise, possible conditions that would be going through my mind would include:

1. Trauma: Is there any evidence of a head injury?
2. Infection: e.g. meningitis, septicaemia — is there any evidence of a skin rash?
3. Neurological: e.g. post-ictal, subarachnoid haemorrhage, space-occupying lesion
4. Toxicological: e.g. salicylates, tricyclic antidepressants, alcohol, glue, anticonvulsants, lead
5. Metabolic: e.g. hypo/hyperglycaemia, Reye's syndrome, Addisonian crisis

In my initial *examination* I would look for a Medic Alert bracelet, evidence of head or neck injury, a rash, pneumothorax, tense abdomen, palpable bladder and I would perform a thorough examination of the neurology. I would look specifically at pupil size and reaction to light, fundoscopy, evidence of nystagmus, signs of meningism, presence or absence of a gag reflex, corneal reflex, tone, reflexes and plantar responses of the limbs and finally calculate a Glasgow coma score.

If by now I was no nearer to a cause, I would undertake several basic investigations: blood glucose, FBC, U&Es, LFTs, Ca and Mg, urine and blood toxicology, arterial blood gases. If there is any suggestion of trauma I would cross-match and save 10 ml of clotted blood, leaving a good i.v. line in situ.

Whilst these investigations are being carried out, I would undertake a more detailed examination and try to obtain further information from relatives. Transfer to ITU is *mandatory* without delay and subsequent investigation would depend upon the cause. These could include head CT scan and involvement of the neurosurgeons if intracranial pathology is suspected, lumbar puncture if there is definitely no raised intracranial pressure, serum ammonia, blood cultures, etc. Insertion of a nasogastric tube and a urinary bladder catheter must be carried out early. Obtaining the patient's medical records may be very enlightening!

Diabetic ketoacidosis

Q. Tell me about your management of diabetic ketoacidosis.

Diabetic ketoacidosis (DKA) is a life-threatening condition of uncontrolled hyperglycaemia associated with ketonuria. It can be the presentation of a new diabetic but more commonly occurs in a known diabetic who has lost normoglycaemic control. I would like to divide management into immediate and more long-term problems.

1. *Immediate*
First, it is necessary to confirm the diagnosis and exclude other possibilities. These would include salicylate ingestion, acute and chronic renal failure, acute gastroenteritis and acute pancreatitis. All of these could present with hyperglycaemia and dehydration and so initial investigation must include tests as mentioned below to exclude these in the unwell child.

Once done, there are five basic problems in DKA:

— dehydration
— hyperglycaemia
— acidosis
— electrolyte disturbance
— causation of the DKA

Dehydration. This is the most important problem that requires immediate attention. The best way to assess the degree of dehydration (usually >10%) is to weigh the patient on admission and compare with a known weight when the child was last well. If the child is shocked or unconscious, he/she requires a rapid infusion of 0.9% saline or PPF/HAS i.v. at 20 ml/kg over 30 minutes. This in itself should produce a dramatic effect on conscious level. Correction of dehydration should then take place over the next 36–48 hours and *deficit + maintenance* is given as isotonic saline, changing to 4% dextrose/0.18% saline once the blood sugar is below 14 mmol/l.

Hyperglycaemia. This is corrected by means of an insulin infusion, running initially at 0.05 U/kg/h intravenously and aiming for a fall in blood glucose of 5 mmol/l/h maximum.

Acidosis. This is assessed by blood gas analysis and usually corrects itself on rehydration and insulin administration. The use of sodium bicarbonate is controversial and is potentially more harmful than beneficial as it can: exacerbate cerebral oedema ($HCO_3 + H^+ \rightleftharpoons H_2O + CO_2$; HCO_3 diffuses slowly through the blood–brain barrier, but CO_2 is readily diffusable, therefore worsening cerebral acidosis and consequent cerebral oedema may occur.); produce hypokalaemia (by pushing K^+ into the cells); and predispose to lactic acidosis.

Electrolyte disturbance. Hyperkalaemia on presentation rapidly changes to hypokalaemia on initiation of treatment and therefore necessitates:

— ECG monitoring
— regular (2–3 hourly initially) serum K+ measurement
— early administration of potassium supplementation to the rehydration solution

Causation of the DKA. Often a child who is unwell with an infection will stop taking their insulin. It is therefore important to look for a focus of infection such as UTI, pneumonia and gastroenteritis. On arrival, when taking initial blood samples, I would include serum glucose, FBC, U&Es, bicarbonate, blood cultures, throat swab, urine for ketones and microbiology, arterial blood gas analysis and save serum.

If the child is unconscious he/she requires care on the ITU. Nasogastric tube insertion is necessary as well as strict monitoring of the urine output, although usually urinary bladder catheterisation is not required. Once the child starts to take fluids and food orally and there is no longer ketonuria, I would revert to his/her normal insulin regimen and discontinue the i.v. fluids.

2. *Long term.*

It is essential to continue education of the child and family to ensure that DKA does not occur again. Reiteration that insulin therapy should never be stopped and early referral to hospital should the child become unwell is advised. Continuing support via outpatients and the community liasion sister is appropriate.

Anaphylaxis

Q. How would you deal with anaphylaxis in general practice?

Anaphylaxis, although rare, is most likely to occur in a GP surgery with immunisation. Between 1978 and 1989 there were 118 reported anaphylactic reactions to immunisations. The steps I would go through for resuscitation are:

1. Lie the patient down in the left lateral position and insert an airway if unconscious
2. Administer 1 in 1000 deep i.m. adrenaline:

   0.05 ml if < 1 year old
   0.1 ml if 1 year old
   0.2 ml if 2 years old
   Maximum 0.5 ml

3. Give face mask oxygen ± CPR
4. Get the patient to hospital and admit for overnight observation
5. Give chlorpheniramine 2.5–5 mg i.v. and hydrocortisone 100 mg i.v.
6. Repeat the i.m. doses of adrenaline up to a maximum of three times
7. Report the reaction to the Committee on Safety of Medicines and avoid subsequent doses of the vaccination

Iron poisoning

Q. A child of 18 months is brought to casualty having been found with a bottle of his mother's iron tablets. What would you do?

I would quickly assess the child, looking for signs of impending shock such as tachycardia, sweating and hypotension, which are due to gastrointestinal haemorrhage. As with all emergencies, I would make sure the child is able to protect his airway, is breathing normally and has good circulation before proceeding. I would question the mother to try to establish how many tablets were in the bottle and whether any were found on the floor. If there is uncertainty as to whether any tablets had been taken and the child is well, I would arrange for an erect chest X-ray, since this may show the ingested tablets.

If it seems likely that tablets have been taken, it is important to try and clear the stomach to prevent absorption. In a well child, it may be possible to induce emesis by giving 15 ml of ipecac with a drink. The dose may be repeated if necessary. 95% of children will vomit with the method. If the child is unco-operative or has impaired consciousness, a gastric lavage is necessary after securing the airway. An experienced paediatric anaesthetist is required. Venous access should be obtained. I would insert a large orogastric tube and aspirate the stomach contents with the child in the semi-prone position. Lavage can then be performed with a large volume of warmed normal saline until the solution aspirated is clear. If tablets are present in the stomach, desferrioxamine solution should be instilled to chelate the iron prior to removal of the orogastric tube. Once more an X-ray will establish whether any tablets have been retained. I would measure serum iron levels which may be high, but the level does not correlate well with the severity of intoxication. Total iron-binding capacity is useful to indicate how much of the iron is free. The white cell count and blood glucose may be raised. Metabolic acidosis also occurs.

Symptoms of iron poisoning in the first few hours include nausea, vomiting, diarrhoea and abdominal pain due to gut irritation. Gut haemorrhage may occur, presenting as haematemesis, rectal bleeding or shock. I would give colloid if signs of shock occur. Whole blood should be ordered and large volumes may be required. Intravenous desferrioxamine infusion (15 mg/kg/h) should be started if the child is shocked or has reduced consciousness. It must be given slowly to prevent hypotension. Desferrioxamine produces a reddish-brown colour in the urine when iron is chelated, therefore the infusion could be stopped when the urine becomes clear. Alternatively, it can be continued until the serum iron levels are reduced.

The child who has accidentally ingested iron should be admitted to hospital for observation. If a substantial amount of iron has been absorbed before treatment is started, there is a risk of deterioration 12–48 hours after ingestion. There may be shock, metabolic acidosis, acute renal failure and hepatocellular necrosis causing death. Fluid balance should be carefully monitored and peritoneal dialysis considered if anuria occurs.

A further complication of iron poisoning starts weeks after ingestion if gastrointestinal bleeding or erosions are present. The child may present with high intestinal obstruction due to strictures secondary to corrosion. I would warn the parents to contact a doctor if the child has recurrent vomiting.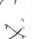

It is important to remind the parents, when the child leaves hospital, that they should keep all medicines and toxic substances locked away. I would also inform the family health visitor so that she can visit and advise on safety in the home.

Stridor

Q. A 2-year old boy is brought to casualty with marked inspiratory stridor. What would your management be?

It is important to establish quickly whether the child has *epiglottitis*. In an effort to gain the confidence of the child, I would talk to his parents with the child sat on their knee. I would ask whether the stridor was of sudden onset and if there had been any prodromal features, such as cough, runny nose or fever. These symptoms are suggestive of viral croup and their absence may be indicative of epiglottitis.

Without disturbing the child, I would observe for cyanosis, drooling of saliva, suprasternal recession and agitation or drowsiness. A child with epiglottitis may be most comfortable sitting upright and immobile. He would be pale and look toxic, with poor peripheral circulation. If after this brief assessment, I felt that epiglottitis was likely, I would contact an experienced paediatric anaesthetist and inform an ENT surgeon, in case a tracheostomy becomes necessary. It is essential not to distress the child, but if he is cyanosed I would give an oxygen mask, with high-flow oxygen, to his mother to hold.

On arrival of the anaesthetist, I would prefer to transfer the child to an ITU where gas induction can be performed in a controlled setting and a tracheal swab taken at the same time. Once the child has been intubated, I would cannulate a vein, take blood cultures and give high-dose cefotaxime until sensitivities of the organism are known.

If I am confident that the child does not have epiglottitis, I would consider other causes of acute stridor such as:

— acute laryngotracheitis
— bacterial tracheitis
— recurrent croup
— foreign body inhalation
— smoke inhalation
— retropharyngeal abcess
— diptheria
— angioneurotic oedema

In all cases, oxygen should be given as required to maintain good saturations on the pulse oximeter. Humidified air is not usually of benefit. The situation needs to be dealt with *calmly*, since any distress will worsen the stridor. A foreign body needs urgent removal. This may be done with Magill's forceps if visible in the larynx, but may need bronchoscopy. Adrenaline and antihistamines should be given promptly if there is a history or signs of allergy. Severe stridor for any cause may require a period of ventilation on clinical grounds. These include a rapidly rising respiratory or pulse rate. Temporary relief may be possible using nebulised adrenaline solution, but these patients need careful observation for fatigue and hypoxia.

Paediatric resuscitation

Q. Tell me about basic resuscitation of the infant and young child in the community?

Unlike adults, cardiac arrest in infancy and childhood is rarely due to primary cardiac disease. It is usually due to hypoxia, either from primary respiratory disease, respiratory depression due to neurological disease or hypotension. By the time myocardial damage is sufficient to cause cardiac arrest, there has already been a period of hypoxia and acidosis.

After the age of 1 year, the most common cause of death is trauma. Early deaths due to trauma happen within minutes, are due to severe injuries and may not be preventable. However, a second group of children die within hours and these deaths are due to circulatory insufficiency, respiratory failure and raised intracranial pressure. It is this group of children who benefit most from early intervention. Training of the general public in basic life support should improve the outcome in these children.

As with adult resuscitation, the basic technique starts with *airway protection*, *breathing*, then *circulation*.

Anatomically the *airway* of a child depends on age. The infant has a relatively large head and a prominent occiput, so when supine the neck is already flexed. Since the trachea is short and soft, over-extension of the neck will cause tracheal compression. When confirmed that a child is not breathing, by looking and feeling for breath over the face, the rescuer should call for help. The head should then be tilted back gently with one hand on the forehead, with the fingers of the other hand under the chin, lifting upwards. If the child has had a head or neck injury the head tilt should be avoided. The finger-sweep technique should also be avoided, since the soft palate is easily damaged. The tongue is proportionately larger in the infant, which may displace posteriorly and cause obstruction. Ideally, an oropharyngeal airway should be inserted. In older children, hypertrophy of the adenoids may also contribute to airway obstruction.

Once the airway is secured, *breathing* should commence. Outside hospital, this is done by opening the mouth slightly and the rescuer covering the mouth and nose of an infant, or the mouth of an older child with the nose pinched, with his/her mouth and slowly exhaling five times. The chest will be seen to rise if the airway is patent. The position of head tilt and chin lift should be altered if this is not the case.

When five rescue breaths have been done, *circulation* should be assessed. In an older child, the carotid artery can be identified. In a younger child or the infant, it is easier to feel the brachial or femoral pulse. If the pulse is absent for 5 seconds, cardiac massage is required. The precordial thump is not recommended in children, since cardiac arrhythmia is an uncommon cause of arrest and damage to the chest wall is more likely.

The child should be flat on his/her back on a hard surface. The technique of compression depends on the size of the child. The infant has a lower heart and compression should be at one finger breadth below the nipple line. Compression can be either with two fingers or by encircling the chest with the hands and compressing smoothly with both thumbs, avoiding compressing the ribs directly. The depth of each compression should be about 2 cm. In a small child, the compression should be down 3 cm with the heel of one hand, one finger breadth above the xiphisternum. In an older child, compression should be down 4 cm, two finger breadths above the xiphisternum with both hands.

A rate of five compressions to one ventilation should be maintained however many rescuers are available. The resting heart rate of a child is higher than the adult, so the cycle rate should be 20 per minute. The emergency services must be contacted.

Some children will start breathing spontaneously after initial resuscitation, so the rescuer needs continually to reassess the situation and stop resuscitation when appropriate.

More advanced life support can take place when the emergency services arrive.

Status epilepticus

Q. Casualty calls to tell you that a 6-year-old girl who has been fitting for 30 minutes is on her way in the ambulance. What would you do?

I would ask that the girl be transferred immediately to the resuscitation room and I would go straight to casualty. Once there, I would ensure that oxygen and suction are readily available and I would prepare equipment for inserting an intravenous line and taking blood. I would arrange for diazepam and other anticonvulsants to be ready to draw up.

On arrival of the patient, I would quickly assess her state and make sure that she has a *patent airway*. This is sometimes difficult as the child may have a clenched jaw, but I would try to clear the mouth of secretions with suction and insert an oropharyngeal airway. I would then give *100% oxygen* by face mask, since oxygen consumption is increased up to five times during status epilepticus. I would ask for a saturation monitor to be put on.

I would then assess the girl quickly to confirm that she is having a convulsion and, if so, what type. In a prolonged fit such as this, my priority would be to stop the fit promptly with short-acting anticonvulsants. My first drug of choice would be *diazepam*. I would ask the parents whether she has had any drugs already, since she may have been given rectal diazepam at home. I prefer to give i.v. diazepam if venous access is easily obtainable. It may be necessary, however, to give the diazepam rectally.

In my experience most parents will stay by their child and I would talk to them while treating their daughter. I would ask whether the girl is a known epileptic and, if so, establish which medications she is on and whether they have been recently reduced. If not known to have fits, I would ask about current febrile illnesses and establish if there are any symptoms suggestive of meningitis. Febrile convulsions are very common in children, but usually start at an earlier age, and prolonged fits are infrequent. I would enquire about a history of trauma and look quickly for bruising. If no other cause is apparent, I would ask about medicines or potential poisons in the house.

While inserting the intravenous line, I would take blood to check blood glucose, calcium, magnesium, sodium, pH and a FBC. I would also do a blood culture if she had a history of fever. Other investigations can wait until the convulsion has stopped.

I would expect the diazepam to be effective within 5–10 minutes. If the fit continues I would give a further dose of diazepam slowly. The side-effects of diazepam, particularly respiratory depression, are more likely after repeated doses and respiratory arrest is a risk.

If there is still no response to diazepam, I would use rectal *paraldehyde* mixed in equal proportions with arachis oil. Paraldehyde can be given intramuscularly, but this is very painful. I have found that paraldehyde works quickly with no respiratory depression and is effective for a longer period of time.

If still fitting, I would give the girl a loading dose of intravenous *phenytoin* over 20 minutes, unless she already uses phenytoin at home. She should be on a cardiac monitor while it is being given, since it may produce cardiac arrhythmias and hypotension.

In the rare case that the convulsion continues, I would transfer the girl to ITU and start a *chlormethiazole* infusion. At this stage, I would consider ventilation after general anaesthetic and muscle relaxants have been given.

When the seizures stop, I would consider whether further investigations are warranted, such as toxicology screen, ammonia, metabolic screen and a cranial CT scan. I would be reluctant to perform a lumbar puncture after such a long fit and I would give antibiotics until meningitis can be safely excluded.

After such a prolonged fit, I would consider fluid restriction to 60% of the normal requirement, in order to prevent cerebral oedema. It may be necessary to give dexamethasone or mannitol if signs of raised intracranial pressure are present.

It is important to remember that complications of status epilepticus are usually due to hypoxia and this must be avoided by giving adequate oxygenation. The temporal horns are particularly vulnerable to ischaemic insult and temporal lobe epilepsy is well described after prolonged status epilepticus. Irreversible neurological handicap may occur after 60 minutes of fitting, so prompt action in casualty with team work is essential.

Status asthmaticus

Q. What is your strategy for management of status asthmaticus?

Asthma results in 40–50 deaths a year in the paediatric population and this number is stubbornly high despite the introduction of a vast array of anti-asthma medications. All too often a child is on inappropriate treatment at home that is ineffective or minimally so with unclear or conflicting instructions for management of acute exacerbations of asthma. A child with asthma can deteriorate rapidly and be in extremis before the medical services are contacted but with appropriate education no child need ever die of his/her asthma.

For a child brought to the hospital with status asthmaticus (i.e. continued respiratory distress with asthma despite anti-asthma medication), I would administer nebulised β_2-agonists with oxygen as soon as possible whilst monitoring heart and respiratory rate and oxygen saturations. Bearing in mind that all that wheezes is not asthma, I would ascertain the facts about the episode of respiratory distress and about previous history of wheeze. Other conditions that merit thought include bronchiolitis, inhalation of foreign body, epiglottitis, smoke inhalation, volatile substance abuse, tracheitis and angioedema. These conditions will require an alternative investigative and managerial plan of action.

If there is little or no clinical and symptomatic improvement on completion of the nebuliser, I would repeat giving continuous face-mask oxygen, insert an i.v. cannula and admit the child to the high dependency unit. In a younger child (<2 years of age). I would also try nebulised ipratoprium bromide. The child requires 24 hour ECG and oxygen saturation monitoring.

The next line of action is contentious and currently a source of research and audit. In my hospital, the child is given i.v. hydrocortisone (4 mg/kg 6 h) and if there is no significant improvement with β_2-agonists, an i.v. aminophylline infusion is set up to continue alongside regular intermittent β_2-agonist nebulisation. I would carry out arterial blood gas sampling and analysis in the more unwell child — if PCO_2 <60 and PO_2 >60 in 40% oxygen, I would continue with the above and review regularly. If PCO_2 >60 or rising rapidly and/or PO_2 <60 in 40% oxygen, I would consider i.v. terbutaline or salbutamol. At any stage, if the child is very dyspnoeic, cyanosed or becoming tired, ventilation with full paralysis and sedation may be required. This fortunately is not a common occurrence but necessitates the skills of a paediatric anaesthetist.

Points of contention in this management include the questionable value of i.v. aminophylline infusions. In less unwell cases, it may offer very little extra, but in very dyspnoeic children it may have some beneficial effect and may just prevent ventilation.

The use of continuous nebuliser β_2-agonists and oral steroids has been suggested as being more effective (i.e. shorter admission time, quicker symptomatic and clinical relief) than intermittent β_2-agonists, i.v. hydrocortisone and i.v. aminophylline. Although the theory is good and very sick children may tolerate a face mask satisfactorily, the less unwell child will object vehemently to having nebulised medication continuously. Aminophylline still has a role in developing countries in the treatment of asthma because of its availability and 'cheapness' compared to β_2-agonists.

Long-term management

Any child who is admitted to hospital with status asthmaticus requiring HDU or ICU care should only be discharged once symptoms are controlled, anti-asthma medication is reviewed and clear written instructions are given to the carers should the child have further exacerbations. There should be 'open access' for 'brittle' asthmatics who:

1. Do not respond to their anti-asthma treatment at home
2. Have only very short-lived relief of symptoms with their treatment, i.e. requiring β_2-agonists every 2–3 hours

REFERENCES

British Thoracic Society Guidelines on the management of asthma 1993 Thorax 48 (suppl): S1–S24

Mackenzie S 1994 Aminophylline in the hospital treatment of children with acute asthma. Br Med J May : 1384

Singh M et al 1993 Continuous nebulised salbutamol and oral once a day prednisolone in status asthmaticus. Arch Dis Child 69: 416–418

A sinister headache

Q1. You have a 14-year-old in outpatients, referred by his GP, with a 2-month history of headaches and nausea. He is accompanied by his mother. What would you do?

Headaches in children are a frequent reason for referral to both general paediatric and paediatric neurology clinics and although usually of a non-serious nature, occasionally have underlying life-threatening disease as their cause. The immediate tasks are:

1. To take an accurate history and examination geared to the possible causes of this problem
2. To decide upon the extent of investigation that is appropriate to be confident there is no serious pathology
3. For the majority of cases which may be classed as 'non-structural' headache, to decide upon the best management

I would consider the possible causes of chronic or recurrent headache and tailor my history and examination to look for the appropriate features. Thus, the main conditions which would pass through my mind in the first instance are:

— psychogenic or tension headache
— migraine
— raised intracranial pressure
— systemic hypertension
— referred headache
— substance abuse
— depression

When I come to examine this child, I would pay particular attention to his blood pressure and pulse and his neurological system, especially the pupils, the fundi, the long tracts, including the plantar response and the tests of co-ordination. I would also examine local areas for possible referred headache such as his ears, eyes for visual acuity, oral cavity and cervical spine. I would plot his growth chart and attempt to make some assessment of higher mental function.

Psychogenic or *tension headache* is the commonest cause of headache and is experienced by the majority of people at some time. There may be a long history and the headache is described as severe, continuous and often as a sense of pressure rather than pain. It is frequently bilateral and often felt over the vault and less frequently occipital or frontal. The headache should lack any suspicious features and examination will be entirely normal. Once confident that I am not dealing with structural disease, further investigation is not required. The child may admit to psychological upset such as family tensions, school-related dissatisfaction or bullying. A picture of psychogenic headache may be an 'acceptable' front with which to manifest a diverse range of underlying problems such as low self-esteem, dyslexia, abuse or sexual tensions. To what extent I would probe into these will depend upon the individual case. If necessary, I would interview the mother and child separately and speak to the GP who will have a better knowledge of the family circumstances.

Migraine is common in childhood (5% of school children increasing to 10% in older age groups). The most obvious clue would be a positive family history which I would expect in about 80% of cases. Most children I have seen with this disorder have complained of a unilateral, often frontal or temporal, throbbing headache, although occasionally they have more generalised symptoms. I would enquire about auras including visual aura (such as scintillating scotomata and zigzag lines — so-called 'fortification phenomena'), mesenteric aura (such as nausea or abdominal fullness) or cranial auras (such as transient ataxia or cranial nerve palsies). I would specifically enquire about precipitating factors such as cow's milk, chocolate, cheese, eggs and tartrazine. Again, I would expect an entirely normal physical examination.

The headache of *raised intracranial pressure* is the most important of the 'structural causes' that I would wish to exclude. I would expect this type of headache to occur in a child in a generally worsening or crescendo pattern over weeks or months and often without a previous history of headache. The headache will often be most severe first thing in the morning, and indeed may wake the child, and will often be associated with nausea and vomiting which may be projectile. The headache will then gradually ease during the day although I would enquire about manoeuvres which tend to increase intracranial pressure such as coughing, straining or bending. On examination, I would look for signs of raised intracranial pressure which are bradycardia, systemic hypertension and papilloedema together with any focal neurological defects. However, these may all be absent and I would still undertake a CT brain scan in a patient with a sufficiently worrying history alone. The main causes of intracranial space occupation are a tumour, vascular malformation or a cyst, and headache is the commonest presenting symptom of posterior fossa lesions. However, I would also consider a cerebral abscess and I would therefore enquire about febrile illnesses, ear or sinus infection and known cardiac septal defects. Also, a chronic subdural haematoma can produce this picture and I would therefore ask about any previous head injury.

Headache due to *systemic hypertension* will often follow the pattern of raised intracranial pressure and as well as the blood pressure, I would examine the optic fundi for evidence of chronicity (A–V nipping, flame-shaped haemorrhages, cotton wool spots and, in the most severe form, papilloedema). If the child is hypertensive, I would also look for features of coarctation and renal disease.

There are various diseases of local structures which may present as *referred headache*, including chronic middle ear disease, dental or chronic sinus disease, refractive errors, strabismus and other ocular disease, and I would therefore look for features of these conditions.

Recurrent headache may be a manifestation of *substance abuse* and in this age group this is most likely to be solvent related such as glue sniffing. Again, interviewing the child and the mother separately and telephoning the GP may be the only way of unravelling this hidden cause if I were suspicious of the diagnosis.

Finally, *depression* in childhood often presents as headache and the condition is easily missed if not specifically considered. I would carefully observe the child during the interview to look for signs of a flattened affect and I would also gently enquire about mood swings, episodes of aggression, social withdrawal and sleep pattern. The diagnosis is a serious one as suicide is not uncommon and I would therefore admit the child and enlist the help of a child psychiatrist if I considered this a possibility.

Q2. **OK, I'll stop you there. You go through the process you've described and feel that there are no particular suspicious features. You advise paracetamol 1 g q.d.s and as a form of reassurance, you arrange a FBC and ESR. You arrange for the child to be seen again in a month's time. However, your SHO phones you at 10 pm one evening to inform you that a 14-year-old boy has been admitted in coma. You arrive and find it is the same boy. Tell me what possible causes would go through your mind.**

I would attempt to link his current presentation with his previous history of chronic headache and nausea. I would therefore consider an intracranial space-occupying lesion, such as a tumour which may have bled or caused cerebral herniation, or an arteriovenous malformation which has now bled, a cerebral abscess or an intracranial haematoma. Another strong possibility is substance abuse. However, after ensuring that the initial management of a patient in coma has been undertaken. I would obtain more information about the mode of the child's admission from anyone accompanying the child, the ambulance drivers or the child's GP.

Q3. **Fine. The ambulance drivers tell you that they were called by the neighbours of this child, who lives on a caravan site. They found the child unconscious on the floor at 9.30 pm. They tell you that his mother normally goes to bingo on a Saturday night and that the boy, Colin, is content to study as he has desires to become a doctor. Indeed, they found him slumped at his desk.**

The fact that this child lives on a caravan site is unusual and would make me concerned that this may be linked to his current illness. Substance abuse is unlikely in a boy who was found at his desk. In addition, the fact that my initial detailed history and examination failed to elicit features of raised intracranial pressure makes the possibility of intracranial space occupation unlikely, although not impossible. I would therefore strongly consider the diagnosis of *carbon monoxide poisoning* from an inadequately ventilated fuel burner. This would explain his initial nausea and headaches and also his unexplained coma as, despite the severe hypoxaemia in this condition, the mucous membranes and skin are pink and not cyanosed because of the formation of carboxyhaemoglobin. I would therefore put the child on 100% oxygen by mask and ensure that he was already on a cardiac monitor. I would then arrange blood gases and carboxyhaemoglobin levels. The normal levels are 1–3% and if sufficient to cause coma, I would expect levels in to be in excess of 30–40%.

If carbon monoxide poisoning is confirmed, two indications for considering hyperbaric oxygen therapy are a state of coma or a carboxyhaemoglobin level >40%. However, this would depend upon the distance to the nearest compression chamber and I would contact the Royal Navy and discuss the case with one of their doctors. I would also anticipate cerebral oedema and if necessary give mannitol by i.v. infusion and i.v. dexamethasone. I would also expect a metabolic acidosis which should respond to the correction of the hypoxaemia.

Q4. Good, the diagnosis did in fact turn out to be carbon monoxide poisoning. What do you know about the pathogenesis of carbon monoxide toxicity?

The affinity of carbon monoxide for haemoglobin is approximately 240 times that for oxygen and therefore the symptoms and signs of carbon monoxide poisoning are related to tissue hypoxia despite the fact that arterial oxygen partial pressure may be normal. Carbon monoxide combines with haemoglobin to form carboxyhaemoglobin which has two potentially disastrous effects. As well as reducing total oxygen carrying capacity, the binding of one or more CO molecules induces an allosteric modification in the haemoglobin, resulting in a greater affinity of the haemoglobin molecule for oxygen, i.e. a left shift of the oxygen dissociation curve. Thus, less oxygen is liberated in the tissues and so the degree of tissue hypoxia is far greater than would result from pure loss of oxygen carriage.

Hyponatraemia

Q1. As the on-call paediatric registrar you are called by the surgical registrar to see a 2-year-old boy on a surgical ward who has been found to have a plasma sodium of 120 mmol/l. Tell me how you would manage this situation.

Hyponatraemia is defined as a plasma sodium below 130 mmol/l and is a relatively common problem in paediatric practice. In the situation you have described, I would expect that arming myself with the history, clinical findings and some basic investigations would in most situations allow me to sort out the likely cause.

There are potentially grave complications of this metabolic derangement, most notably *cerebral impairment* and *convulsions* and the likelihood of these will depend upon the rapidity of the fall of the plasma sodium, as well as the absolute level. It is important to unravel the underlying problem and direct treatment accordingly rather than simply considering the plasma sodium alone. Indeed, inappropriate treatment may itself precipitate complications.

Whilst on the phone, I would establish from my surgical colleague that the child is stable and not in need of immediate resuscitation. On arrival, I would briefly confirm that the sample is a genuine one and not one obtained 'upstream' from a drip-arm, which I have found to be a common explanation for this problem (especially in August!). I would also keep in mind the possibility of 'pseudo-hyponatraemia' in hyperlipidaemic or hyperproteinaemic states. This produces measured whole-plasma hyponatraemia with a normal concentration in plasma water and therefore at the cell surface.

I would then obtain a history from the surgical registrar, and from the parents if they are present, the case notes, paying particular attention to the reason for admission and what, if any, surgical procedures had been carried out. I would also enquire about the boy's general health including perinatally (CAH) and his general past medical and surgical history and any recent problems such as diarrhoea or vomiting. Recent medication may be relevant in the case of prolonged steroid therapy or various drugs which may cause inappropriate ADH secretion. I would also ask the surgical registrar to show me the treatment chart and any recent investigations. I would pay particular attention to the input/output chart and calculate the total fluid balance over the past few days and take note of what fluids had been used.

On examining the child, I would pay particular attention to the state of hydration, the pulse and blood pressure and signs of peripheral oedema. I would also look for signs of chronic liver or renal disease and make my own subjective assessment of whether the child looked generally well or unwell.

I normally begin with a few basic investigations which may already be available, including the U&Es, blood glucose, plasma and urine osmolality and sodium concentration. In some situations, the blood gases may be important.

Based upon my examination findings, I normally categorise the hyponatraemia into one of three groups where there is:

1. A state of dehydration
2. Peripheral oedema
3. Clinically normal hydration

This simplifies the assessment and investigation of the possible causes of this boy's hyponatraemia which will in turn guide therapy.

The *dehydrated hyponatraemic* child suggests hypotonic dehydration with disproportionate loss of sodium over water. In this situation, the extracellular fluid is more hypotonic than intracellular fluid which tends to cause fluid shift into cells. This means that there is a serious risk of both cerebral oedema leading to convulsions and a greater degree of shock per unit volume of fluid loss.

Careful questioning of the surgical registrar and the parents should exclude *gastroenteritis* or other cause of *vomiting* or *diarrhoea*. I would also consider other causes of gastrointestinal fluid loss such as *obstruction* or *fistulae* (? Crohn's disease). Losses from the skin due to severe *burns* will again be obvious. In all of these situations, the urinary sodium concentration will be low (below 20 mmol/l) in an attempt to conserve total body sodium.

Other diagnoses that lead to renal loss of hypertonic fluid are:

— adrenal cortical hypofunction
— renal failure (diuretic phase)
— osmolar diuresis in DKA
— primary forms of renal tubular acidosis

A high plasma potassium (above 5.5 mmol/l) would favour the first three. If I found this picture together with a metabolic acidosis and a low or low–normal plasma potassium, I would consider primary renal tubular acidosis as the likely cause.

Both renal failure and DKA should be readily identifiable from my basic investigations. *Adrenal cortical hypofunction* (due to congenital adrenal hyperplasia, prolonged steroid therapy, Addison's disease or fulminating infection) is an often forgotten and easily missed medical emergency which is particularly likely to manifest following the stress of surgery. I may have clues to this diagnosis in the history (neonatal problems in CAH, steroid therapy) and examination (a child that looks unwell with unaccountable hypotension and weakness and, if Addison's disease, pigmentation). I would specifically check the blood sugar to look for complicating *hypoglycaemia*. Additionally, I would be aware of the possibility of prominent GI symptoms being mistaken for gastroenteritis.

If I seriously suspected the diagnosis, especially in the face of the metabolic picture I have already described (or other features such as an elevated urea and hypochloraemic acidosis), I would immediately perform a short *Synacthen test* (take t=0 plasma cortisol, give 250 μg i.v. or i.m. of Synacthen and take t=30 and

60 min plasma cortisol). I would then commence therapy as soon as I had taken the initial bloods and given the Synacthen if the clinical situation was sufficiently urgent. This would comprise i.v. normal saline fluid replacement (20 ml/kg), i.v. hydrocortisone sodium succinate 50 mg followed by 5 mg/kg per 24 hours in six divided doses and correction of hypoglycaemia. Although hydrocortisone is essentially a glucocorticoid, it has sufficient mineralocorticoid activity to make it the drug of choice in the immediate management of both secondary and primary adrenal failure.

The results of the short Synacthen test are not available immediately but are still interpretable even if I have to commence therapy. A normal 2–3 fold increase in plasma cortisol after Synacthen excludes the diagnosis. I would bear in mind that hypotension with hyponatraemia, hyperkalaemia and uraemia may be present in many acute clinical situations as well as in Addisonian crisis. However, it is still appropriate to treat blind if the diagnosis is suspected as there are few complications of this regimen and the consequences of delaying treatment of the condition may be grave.

Q2. Tell me what your thoughts would be if you found this child to be oedematous.

Causes of hyponatraemia with oedema:

— hypoproteinaemic states such as nephrotic syndrome and liver disease (either chronic or fulminant)
— fluid-overload states such as injudicious fluid replacement (especially if dextrose solutions have been used), renal failure and cardiac failure

Once again, a careful history and examination, inspection of the fluid-balance chart and some basic blood and urine investigations should direct me towards the underlying cause. Daily weights (if they had been recorded) may also be very revealing.

Q3. OK, tell me your thoughts if your examination found that the boy was neither dehydrated nor oedematous.

The most important cause of hyponatraemia with clinically normal hydration is the *syndrome of inappropriate ADH secretion (SIADH)*. Children seem particularly likely to show this metabolic reaction and common antecedent causes are respiratory illness, trauma (including surgical) and cerebral disease (such as trauma or infection). It may also be a complication of certain drugs such as opiates, carbamazepine or cytotoxics.

The diagnosis is based on the finding of hyponatraemia with a low plasma osmolality (below 270 mmol/kg) in the face of an inappropriately high urine osmolality or high urine sodium concentration (above 40 mmol/l). This will usually mean a urine: blood osmolality ratio >2 (i.e. a urine osmolality above 500 mmol/kg). However, the diagnosis should still be considered at levels short of this if the urine osmolality is considered to be inappropriately high with respect to the plasma value.

The complications are decreasing conscious level and convulsions which may be dangerously worsened by inappropriate fluid replacement if the condition is not recognised. The best management of SIADH is *fluid restriction to 50% of* normal which will result in slow restoration of plasma sodium and osmolality. In the acutely-ill child, careful use of normal (which in any situation tends to normalise plasma osmolality) or even hypertonic saline, obeying strict regimens, may be justified. This must be done with extreme caution to avoid the cerebral complications or over-rapid correction of plasma osmolality. Rather paradoxically, diuretics such as frusemide are occasionally used to treat SIADH.

Other possible causes of this pattern are mild adrenocortical hypofunction or, again, injudicious fluid replacement. In both of these situations, the urine osmolality will not be inappropriately high.

Pyrexia in a child on long-term steroids

Q. A child who is on long-term steroids attends casualty with a pyrexia of unknown origin. Are there any precautions you would consider?

Corticosteroids are *immunosuppressive* agents and as a result patients on high-dose oral steroids are at an increased risk of overwhelming sepsis. Whether this applies to a lesser extent in those taking inhaled or topical steroids is not fully known. Manifestations of severe infection may be masked by the steroids and so greater caution should be taken with these children. It is important to note that for a period of up to 3 months after stopping high-dose oral steroids, children are considered immunocompromised.

Disseminated chickenpox and measles are of particular concern as they can be fatal in immunocompromised children. Each year around 30 people die of chickenpox and one-third of these are secondary to immunosuppression. A proportion of these are on high-dose steroids. The Committee on Safety of Medicines reports at least a 100-fold increased risk of severe varicella infection if on steroids.

There is no increased risk to children on steroids who have had definite chickenpox or who have adequate antibody titres to varicella zoster. However, in those without adequate titres or no previous history of chickenpox, precautions are necessary:

1. Avoidance of exposure to chickenpox or herpes zoster wherever possible
2. If exposure occurs, passive immunisation with varicella zoster immunoglobin should be carried out within 3 days of exposure
3. If a chickenpox rash develops (and it may not be a prominent feature in these children), a 10-day course of i.v. acyclovir is indicated.

If none of the above applies to this child with PUO, admission may be justified in order to observe for a short time. Throat swab, urine culture and blood culture are worthwhile and a lumbar puncture should be performed if there is any suggestion of disseminated infection.

Finally, with the resurgence of tuberculosis in the UK, this diagnosis must be considered and excluded by chest X-ray, Heaf test, etc.

REFERENCES

Committee on Safety of Medicines 1994 Severe chickenpox associated with systemic corticosteroids. Current problems in pharmaco-vigalance Feb: 1–2

Dowell S F et al 1993 Severe varicella associated with steroid use. Pediatrics 92: 223–228

A child with multiple injuries

Q. What would be your assessment and management for a child brought to casualty with multiple injuries?

Fortunately this is not a common problem, but when encountered it should be dealt with speedily and efficiently and yet extremely thoroughly to maximise the child's opportunity for survival and to prevent morbidity. Regular training sessions and lectures for this eventuality are necessary and attendance of Advanced Paediatric Life Support courses must be recommended to staff who may deal with multiply injured children.

Ideally, some warning of this child's arrival will be given so that relevant medical and nursing staff can be on stand-by in casualty. In the same way as I would deal with an unconscious child, there are four basic steps to assessment and management:

1. Initial assessment
2. Resuscitation
3. Secondary more detailed assessment
4. Definitive care

1. *Initial assessment* involves as always the ABC of resuscitation. Does this child have a patent airway, is he/she breathing and does this child have a normal circulation? Also included in this initial assessment should be a measure of conscious level, pupil reactivity and, very importantly, protection of the cervical spine, on the assumption that damage has occurred until proven otherwise. Any available information from the ambulance crew, the child, family, etc. in attendance should be sought by a third party.

2. *Resuscitation*

   — Airway — jaw thrust, but not head tilt should be carried out and removal of foreign material from the mouth by suction
   — Breathing — intubation and ventilation is necessary if the child does not have spontaneous and adequate respiration following a short period of bag and mask resuscitation with oxygen, but I would seek the skills of a trained paediatric anaesthetist to perform the intubation, unless the situation dictated otherwise
   — Circulation — rapid vascular access is essential in multiply injured children but very often siting of large bore cannulae percutaneously is

technically difficult or impossible. Intraosseus cannulation is easy and reliable. On obtaining access, blood can be taken for haematology, biochemistry and cross-matching. Depending on the clinical situation, appropriate intravenous/intraosseus infusions can be started

Whilst the above procedures are being done, X-rays of the cervical spine, chest and pelvis can be organised, plus any other X-rays deemed appropriate.

Urinary catheterisation and nasogastric tube insertion can be performed at this stage and analgesic administered unless contraindicated.

3. More *detailed assessment* can be carried out once the child is stable, albeit possibly temporarily, hence the need for continued re-assessment of vital signs. A thorough examination from head to toe can identify potential problems that may require surgical or orthopaedic intervention, immediately or at a later date. By this time a history should have been obtained, the child is stable, appropriate investigations have been carried out and the child is ready for transfer to PICU or theatre. The relevant specialities have given their opinions and will know where the child is to go to for continued reassessment. Monitoring of vital signs is an on-going and continuous process and must include pulse, blood pressure, respiratory rate, pupil reaction, urine output, Glasgow coma scale and in my hospital a PRISM score, an indicator of ultimate prognosis.

A persistently screaming infant

Q. What are your thoughts about an infant that is brought to you because of excessive and persistent crying?

Persistent crying in infancy is particularly prevalent in the under 3 month olds and is usually blamed on 'colic'. Characteristically, the crying occurs in the afternoons and evenings and, whatever the parents seem to do, nothing will console their baby. In those babies who are considered by their parents to have excessive crying, objective measurements have confirmed this (an average $3\frac{1}{4}$– $3\frac{3}{4}$ hours vs $2\frac{1}{4}$–$2\frac{1}{2}$ hours per 24 hours for a 'normal' infant).

The main problem for the medical practitioner and for the parents is to differentiate between *organic* and *behavioural* causes. Many proposals for causation of 'colic' have been put forward:

— intestinal dilatation and peristalsis
— cow's milk whey intolerance
— difficult temperament of the baby
— delayed development of the parasympathetic nervous system
— 'jet lag': the transition from a 4-hour feed/sleep pattern to a 24-hour sleep/ wake cycle
— inadequate caring
— parental smoking

There are an equal number of suggested treatments for persistent crying:

— reduction in stimulation of the baby when crying
— carrying the baby around during troublesome periods
— changing from cow's milk based formulae to a hydrolysed casein formula milk
— gentle rocking of the baby in quiet surroundings
— dicyclomine hydrochloride (withdrawn for under 6 month olds because of reported breathing difficulties, seizures and coma)

Very often by the time of referral to hospital, the parents are at the end of their tether. They will have been given conflicting advice about what should and should not be done, all to no effect. Anxiety will be high and in the more severe cases the risk of non-accidental injury must be borne in mind. In such circumstances a period of time in hospital simply to allow parents to catch up on sleep may be justified. The possibility of cow's milk intolerance is probably over estimated, but if there is a strong family history and a subjective relief of symptoms with a change of formula, then this can be an appropriate approach.

For the breast-fed baby, dietary advice for the mother is necessary to exclude the passage of cow's milk products through the breast milk.

The question of degree of stimulation for a baby that is persistently crying is very contradictory. The advice to simply leave a baby crying is extremely difficult for a caring mother to carry through. On the other hand, the mother should not rush to pick up the baby as soon as he/she stirs or cries out as the episode may last only several seconds if left undisturbed. Overfeeding a baby is not a satisfactory solution.

Reassurance is all important for the parents. The infant will 'grow out' of his/her excessive crying, usually by 3 months of age and early weaning may speed resolution. Also reassure that no long-term damage or harm is being done to the infant.

Parents often report increased crying after an infant is given DTPP and Hib vaccinations — this is not a contraindication to subsequent immunisations unless excessive. The incidence of crying is 60% whether it is the 1st, 2nd or 3rd vaccination, and inconsolable crying occurs in 2–3%. Parental advice prior to vaccination should include warning of likely symptoms and signs and the suggestion that paracetamol be administered before subsequent jabs.

REFERENCES

McKenzie S 1991 Troublesome crying infants: effect of advice to reduce stimulation. Arch Dis Child 66: 1416–1420

St Jams-Roberts I 1991 Persistent infant crying. Arch Dis Child 66: 653–655

Verschoor P L et al 1991 Frequent symptoms after DTPP vaccination Arch Dis Child 66: 1408–1412

Paracetamol overdose

Q. How would you manage a child who has taken a significant overdose of paracetamol?

Paracetamol overdose in childhood takes two forms:

1. *Accidental* ingestion of syrups of paracetamol, e.g. Calpol, Disprol, Medised, Salzone, Panadol. This occurs in the infant and toddler because of their naturally inquisitive behaviour and the pleasant taste of these preparations. Care must be taken to ascertain exactly which preparation has been ingested as other drugs may have been incorporated into the syrup, e.g. promethazine contains both Codeine and Aspirin.
2. *Deliberate* ingestion in adolescents, almost always as a cry for help but just occasionally as a serious succide attempt.

The National Poisons Information Service (NPIS) has brought out new guidelines for the management of paracetamol overdose. In all suspected cases of ingestion it is judicious practice to assume the worst and treat rather than delay treatment and waste valuable hours whilst results become available.

In all children who have taken >150 mg/kg (or >5 g in over 12 year olds) or in any child who cannot give an accurate account of things, treatment must be given. The value of >100 mg/kg should be used in children who are taking anticonvulsant medication because of their induction effect upon liver enzymes.

Time of ingestion

1. <4 *hours.* I would give lpecacuanha syrup and, once the child has stopped vomiting, charcoal by mouth. Charcoal is very difficult to get down an unwilling and uncooperative child. Its purpose is to bind with paracetamol and therefore decrease absorption. In the USA, oral methionine is used as the antidote for paracetamol poisoning, rather than N-acetylcysteine. However, charcoal also binds methionine and thereby decreases its efficacy.

2. 4 *hours.* I would take serum for paracetamol levels and, if large amounts of paracetamol have been ingested, consider base-line LFTs and clotting. Serum should be saved for further toxocological investigation if deemed necessary at a later date. I would start treatment with i.v. N-acetylcysteine if serum paracetamol levels are >200 mg/l.

3. 4–8 *hours.* Emptying the stomach is probably ineffective. I would simply measure serum paracetamol levels and start treatment immediately if the

child is 'toxic' (unconscious, vomiting) until the result of the levels becomes available.

4. *8–24 hours.* I would give N-acetylcysteine immediately and continue until the paracetamol levels are back. This antidote can be stopped if the levels turn out to be non toxic.

5. *24–36 hours.* I would start N-acetylcysteine if the history suggested significant paracetamol ingestion. I would then check INR (international normalised ratio), LFTs and plasma paracetamol levels. Antidote would only be considered if the INR was >2, the LFTs were deranged or plasma paracetamol levels were still detectable. INR, LFTs and U&Es need daily checking. Recommendations for referral to a liver unit include:

— INR >2 at 24 hours post ingestion
— INR >4 at 48 hours post ingestion
— INR >6 at 72 hours post ingestion
— elevated creatinine
— evidence of encephalopathy
— hypotension following volume replacement
— metabolic acidosis with pH <7.3

N-acetylcysteine (Parvolex) is made up as an infusion in 5% dextrose:

1. 150 mg/kg over 15 minutes
2. 50 mg/kg over 4 hours
3. 100 mg/kg over 16 hours

N-acetylcysteine can rarely cause anaphylaxis, but this is not a contraindication to treatment in the general paediatric population on admission, whatever time period has elapsed since ingestion.

In those that have deliberately taken paracetamol, referral to the child psychiatry service is important prior to discharge from the paediatric ward. In those that have accidentally ingested paracetamol, the parents should be made aware of the potential dangers of ingestions and preventative advice given, supplemented by educational leaflets. In recurrent 'offenders' social service input may be of benefit.

REFERENCES

Lovejoy et al 1993 Common aetiologies and new approaches to management of poisoning in paediatric practice. Curr Opin Paed 5: (5)

Reye's syndrome

Q. Reye's syndrome is a rare and interesting condition. What can you tell me about it?

Reye's syndrome is a very uncommon illness of acute non-inflammatory encephalopathy and hepatopathy, typically (in at least 90%) preceded by a viral illness, e.g. influenza B, varicella, coxsackie and echovirus. The BPSU has reported a dramatic reduction in annual incidence since the mid 1980s. This follows advice suggesting the avoidance of Aspirin for under 12s as an antipyretic agent. Current incidence is around 15 true reported cases a year.

The diagnosis has to be differentiated from *inborn errors of metabolism* that can present clinically and pathologically as Reye's syndrome. Such conditions include:

— fatty acid oxidation defects, e.g. MCAD/LCAD deficiency
— amino acid disorders, e.g. HMG CoA lyase deficiency
— urea cycle disorders, e.g. OTC deficiency
— mitochondrial electron transfer defects

In every child that presents with a Reye-like illness, detailed investigation must be undertaken to exclude an inborn error of metabolism, i.e. serum ammonia, amino acids, glucose, U&Es, transaminases, urinary organic acids and amino acids, orotic acid excretion, and demonstration of deficient enzyme activity.

Essentially there are four pathological derangements:

1. Raised ICP
2. Hypoglycaemia
3. Coagulopathy
4. Hyperammonaemia

1. *Raised ICP*: this is the most important of the four and may require aggressive treatment. This occurs secondary to cerebral oedema which in turn results from mitochondrial disruption. Cerebral perfusion pressure can be calculated as:

   Mean arterial pressure – intracranial pressure
   and should be maintained above 50 mmHg. This can be achieved, depending on severity, by fluid restriction, osmotic diuretics, hyperventilation and even surgical decompression.

2. *Hypoglycaemia*: this occurs secondary to glycogen depletion. Normoglycaemia is maintained by the administration of 10–20% dextrose i.v.

3. *Coagulopathy*: secondary to thrombocytopenia and hepatopathy. This may necessitate administration of platelets, vitamin K and FFP, respectively.

4. *Hyperammonaemia*: again secondary to hepatopathy. Whether this needs active treatment is controversial but plasmaphoresis and peritoneal dialysis have been advocated by some.

Mortality from this condition is around 40% and is dependent on conscious level at presentation. A grading system can be used, with: grade 1 (lethargic at presentation) almost always gaining full recovery, often with minimal intervention; grade 2 (confusion); grade 3 (light coma); grade 4 (decerebrate rigidity) and grade 5 (flaccidity/decerebrate) who invariably die or are left severely disabled.

Acute abdominal pain

Q. I want you to imagine that you are planning a talk on the assessment of acute abdominal pain in children for a group of local GPs. Tell me the main points which you would like to get across in your talk.

My audience will probably have seen as many children with an acute abdomen as I have and my aim would be to build on their existing experience and highlight a few important or interesting points. I would start by reminding them that there are numerous possible causes of acute abdominal pain in childhood and they will probably have encountered many of these in their clinical practice.

Children, like elderly patients, are deceivers. Simple benign illness may present with a very sick-looking child. More importantly, potentially life-threatening disease may present relatively innocuously without classical signs and trap the unwary clinician.

Most causes are *common* and relatively benign, often being related to viral illness of one form or other and can therefore be safely managed at home. Where doubt remains in the case of a moderately unwell child, a review after 4–6 hours will usually determine whether admission is necessary.

The *age* and *sex* of the child has a major bearing on the assessment. A child under 2 years will be unable to give any meaningful history. In general terms, the threshold for admission of a very young child should be low. Intussusception, for example, should be considered in infants and toddlers (usually 3–24 months) with screaming attacks. The child will usually have been unwell for 1–2 days and there may have been the passage of the classic bloody mucus stool of redcurrant jelly appearance. This is, however, a late sign and not invariable. The typical sausage mass in the right upper quadrant is often difficult to feel. I would stress that in between spasms of pain, these children may appear remarkably well. Intussusception and obstruction due to inguinal herniae are both more common in boys. Similarly, it is vital to examine the testes of any boy who presents with acute abdominal pain to exclude torsion.

Conversely, some conditions which should be considered in older girls include dysmenorrhoea, mid-cycle ovulation pain (mittelschmertz), torsion or rupture of an ovarian cyst and pelvic inflammatory disease. In some situations, it may even be appropriate to consider an ectopic pregnancy (pelvic pain with or without vaginal bleeding, shoulder pain or fainting attacks in a girl who may or may not admit that she has missed a period).

Further relevant aspects of the history include recent and past health, vomiting, diarrhoea or constipation, urinary symptoms (in a baby, is he/she wetting more often or crying with micturition?), polydipsia and the appearance of any rash.

The GP may have vital knowledge of the family which would suggest a variety of diagnoses such as gastroenteritis, non-organic abdominal pain (stressful situations at home or at school), recurrent abdominal pain (family history of migraine) or even clues to NAI.

It goes without saying that a careful thorough *examination* of the whole child is essential. The general appearance of the child in between episodes of pain should be assessed but I would stress again that this can be misleading. Certain conditions which may present with an acute abdomen are renown to cause diagnostic confusion:

Mesenteric adenitis and infectious mononucleosis	Examine for an upper respiratory illness and signs of lymphadenopathy. Splenic rupture can (rarely) take place spontaneously or with minimal trauma in IM
Pneumonia (especially right lower lobe)	Careful examination of the chest — look carefully for tachypnoea which may be the only sign
Henoch-Schönlein purpura	Look carefully at the buttocks, thighs and ankles for the petechial rash which usually but not always precedes the pain
Diabetic ketoacidosis	Tachypnoea with sighing respiration, pear-drops smell to the breath and a diffusely painful but minimally tender abdomen
Sickle cell disease	Always consider in children from appropriate ethnic groups
Hernial and genital disease	Always carefully examine the hernial orifices and genitalia

Urinalysis and *urine culture* should always be carried out in any child with an acute abdomen. Urinalysis may point to a UTI, HSP, DKA or sickle cell disease as the cause. Significant ketosis without glycosuria may confirm the clinical suspicion of an unwell, dehydrated child.

I would remind the audience that UTI in childhood carries far more implications than in adults and therefore an MSU should always be sent. Parents should be instructed to obtain a 'clean-catch' specimen from babies as bag specimens are often misleading. If this shows a genuine positive result, further investigation is indicated (regardless of the sex of the child).

I would remind my colleagues that *appendicitis* can be an extremely difficult diagnosis to make in childhood and once again GPs will probably know that children are similar to patients at the other extreme of age in this respect. Constipation is usual but an inflamed pelvic appendix may irritate the rectum and cause the passage of loose stool which may be misinterpreted as the diarrhoea of gastroenteritis. Soaring pyrexias should *not* be expected; the temperature rarely exceeds 38.5°C unless perforation has occurred. 'Apyrexial appendicitis' is a well recognised entity in children.

The appendix is longer and thinner in the under 4s. Therefore, although appendicitis is uncommon in this age group, it is more likely to perforate and present with generalised peritonitis. Classical features are often absent and general non-specific tenderness plus a reluctance to be examined may be the only signs. As with any paediatric examination, a playful, unhurried approach is vital. Examining teddy or using the diaphragm of the stethoscope to elicit tenderness are useful 'tricks'. Asking older children to hop and indicate the site of any pain is sometimes a good test for localised peritonitis.

Tips

- Sometimes the examiners will test your mental agility as well as experience by using an unusual angle such as planning a talk. Another example is giving advice to a learned non-paediatric friend in a pub, e.g. on how to protect their young one from SIDS.

- Use the situation to your advantage! Do as they say and forget that you are facing two membership examiners. Pretend that they are two GP trainee friends who have asked you to educate them! Show flare and style as well as demonstrating that you have hands-on experience of assessing a child with an acute abdomen.

Apnoea

Q. A 3-month-old infant is brought to casualty with a history of stopping breathing. What would you do?

I would first assess whether the infant was breathing on arrival. If not, I would resuscitate the child by protecting the airway, then giving oxygen using a bag and mask system and starting cardiac massage if required. Intubation would be necessary if breathing is not quickly re-established.

If the infant is breathing normally, I would put a saturation monitor on to judge whether oxygen is required. I would talk to the parents as soon as possible to find out exactly what happened. I would ask what colour the child seemed, whether he/she was floppy or stiff, whether he/she had been sleeping or awake at the time, what position he/she was in and if he/she had recently been fed. Although it is always difficult to remember how long a serious event like this lasted, I would ask the parents to estimate how long they think their child stopped breathing for. I would also ask if they noticed any chest wall movement during the episode as the child may have had shallow breathing or at a reduced rate. In order to assess the severity of the episode, I would ask what form of resuscitation was needed to start the baby breathing again and how long it took for the baby to get back to normal.

Apnoeas may be classified as obstructive, central or mixed. They may be due to a specific and treatable disorder, but in at least 50% of cases, no cause is found. The most common causes are:

1. *Infection:* particularly bronchiolitis due to respiratory syncitial virus and pertussis infection. Other infections which may cause apnoea are septicaemia, meningitis and occasionally UTI. Enteroviruses, such as Coxsachie and Echo, may also cause hypotonia and collapse in the young infant.
2. *Upper airway obstruction:* either due to structural abnormalities, e.g. in Pierre–Robin syndrome and Down's syndrome, or due to blockage with secretions in upper respiratory infection in narrow airways.
3. *Seizures:* convulsions may present at any age but classic tonic–clonic convulsions are less common in this age group.
4. *Gastro-oesophageal reflux:* common in infancy. Reflux of stomach contents may stimulate the laryngeal chemoreceptor reflex causing apnoea. The actual volume of fluid refluxing is probably not as important.
5. *Cardiac disease:* arrhythmias, e.g. supraventricular tachycardia and congenital heart disease, may cause cyanosis and collapse.
6. *Trauma:* it is important to exclude trauma as sub-dural haemorrhage may cause apnoea.

Less commonly, apnoea may be due to:

1. Anaemia: this may occur if the packed cell volume is 0.25.
2. Central nervous system tumours.
3. Central hypoventilation syndromes: known as 'Ondine's curse'.
4. Intrapulmonary shunting.
5. Metabolic disorders, e.g. hypoglycaemia.

Apnoea may also occur if the infant is too hot or has been left lying face down.

Immediate *investigations* should include a blood gas. This will help to find out how severe the apparent life-threatening event was. Metabolic acidosis may, however, be due to an underlying metabolic disease. I would also check the blood glucose, electrolytes and a FBC. I would take blood and urine for culture and consider a lumbar puncture. If the history suggests a respiratory cause for the apnoea, I would arrange a nasopharyngeal aspirate for viruses and a pernasal swab for pertussis. Chest X-ray and electrocardiogram may be appropriate. In some cases skull X-ray and cranial ultrasound are warranted. An EEG may be helpful, but could be left until the infant is fully recovered, since the hypoxic event will have an effect on the EEG and make epileptic activity difficult to interpret.

I would admit the child to hospital for observation of respiratory rate and saturations. If no further episodes occurred and no cause was found, I would instruct the parents in basic life support. I would not offer an apnoea alarm unless the parents were very keen to use one, since they have not been shown to influence mortality.

The prognosis for the child who has an apparent life-threatening event such as this is uncertain. A minority will have serious neurological damage due to this initial event and for these the prognosis is poor. The risk of further episodes obviously depends on the cause, but for those with ideopathic apnoeas requiring resuscitation, a third will have a further episode. These mainly seem to occur within 2 weeks of the first.

Tips

■ The examiners do not want you to recite a long list of causes. This is just a helpful list for revision purposes.

■ The best approach is to suggest an investigation and then explain why you would do it, e.g. "I would do a chest X-ray to look at the size of the heart and for evidence of consolidation since respiratory infection and congenital heart disease are common causes of apnoea".

Hypertensive emergencies

Q1. A 5-year-old boy is sent to your A&E department by his GP with a severe headache. On arrival, his blood pressure is recorded at 180/118 mmHg. Tell me what you would do.

I would expect a child of 5 years to have a resting blood pressure of around 95/60 mmHg and I would confirm this by looking at centile charts for normal ranges. A blood pressure of 180/118 mmHg would tie in with his symptoms but I would first re-check the recording. I would sit the child comfortably or lying flat for at least 3 minutes and if the child is agitated, I would attempt, with the help of the parents, to settle him. Having placed the sphygmomanometer at the level of the heart and using the widest cuff which can be applied to the right upper arm (covering at least $\frac{2}{3}$ of it), I would repeat the recording at least twice.

If I confirmed a similarly high BP, I would put an automatic oscillometry 'Dinamap' recorder on the child so that I had continued sequential measurements. I would then look into the child's fundi with an ophthalmoscope whilst at the same time taking a brief history from the parents. I would be looking for signs *of acute end-organ damage* such as flame-shaped haemorrhages and papilloedema which would confirm my suspicions that this boy has severe accelerated or *'malignant' hypertension*. As the term suggests, this implies a condition which, if untreated, will lead to death within a few days or weeks.

Q2. Fine. Let's assume that you have confirmed this. How would you treat this condition acutely.

I would secure peripheral venous access and either initially or during therapy, consider a CVP line dictated by the child's condition. CVP monitoring may be important during therapy as these patients may be hypo-, hyper- or normovolaemic. I would also assess the vital signs, urine output, pupils and fundi regularly. In accelerated hypertension, relative or absolute hypotension may be as dangerous as hypertension because of the risk of cerebral hypoperfusion and subsequent infarction. A gradual *controlled reduction in blood pressure* is therefore the aim of treatment of accelerated hypertension. I would calculate the desired fall in blood pressure and aim for $\frac{1}{3}$ of this to be achieved over not <6 hours. The remaining $\frac{2}{3}$ of the reduction should then take place over the ensuing 24 hours.

Emergency treatment of severe hypertension traditionally involved intravenous labetalol or sodium nitroprusside. More recent reports, however, suggest that sublingual *nifedipine* is effective and has the advantage of a safe and easy route of administration. I would begin at a dose of 0.2 mg and, if necessary, work up to a maximum of 0.5 mg every 2 hours. Nifedipine by this route has a speed of onset of activity of within half an hour and should last between 3 and 12 hours. The main difficulty lies in the fact that the solution has to be obtained from a 5 or 10 mg nifedipine capsule using a syringe with a narrow gauge needle and that a calculated volume has to be administered.

If this is ineffective, I would next use *hydrallazine* at a dose of 0.2 mg/kg by i.v. infusion over at least 20 minutes. I would go up to 0.8 mg/kg and repeat the dose up to 1 hourly if necessary. In resistant cases, I would consider i.v. diazoxide, labetalol (contraindicated in asthma) or sodium nitroprusside. If the child developed a tachycardia during the administration of vasodilator drugs, I would commence an oral β-blocker (providing the child is not asthmatic or in heart failure), such as propranolol starting at 1.0 mg/kg/24 hours.

Tips

- This is a good example of listening carefully and answering the question that is asked. Clearly, the situation demands a full assessment including various investigations both acutely and longer term. However, treatment of the child acutely is asked for and it is this problem which you are required to address.

- To what extent you must know doses is contentious and probably depends heavily on the individual examiner; as a minimum, it is worth knowing first-line emergency drug regimens.

Intraosseous infusion

Q1. You will know that the intraosseous route is infrequently employed but nevertheless is an important route for vascular access. Tell me about it.

The intraosseous route is an extremely valuable and generally safe method of obtaining rapid and reliable access to the vascular bed in children in critical situations. It is usually used when more conventional routes cannot be readily secured, such as in cardiorespiratory arrest, major trauma, massive sepsis, shock and status epilepticus.

Delays in obtaining vascular access have been reported in about 25% of paediatric emergencies and all paediatricians need to be familiar with this technique.

The route employs accessing the bone marrow of long bones which drains via the sinusoids and central venous channels to exit the bone via emissary veins and enter the general circulation. It has been shown that absorption from bone marrow is excellent and systemic drug levels produced in emergency situations are similar to those achieved with central venous administration. Therefore, once secured, this route is preferable to the endotracheal administration of resuscitation drugs (Hapnes & Robertson 1992). In older children, the highly vascular red marrow is gradually replaced by less vascular yellow marrow and so the technique is only used in children under 7 years. It is especially useful in the resuscitation of babies.

There are specially designed intraosseous needles but if not rapidly available spinal needles can be used instead. I would use 20–16 gauge for the under 2s and 16–12 gauge for older children. I would choose the anteromedial surface of the proximal tibia at a point 2–3 cm distal to the tibial tuberosity to avoid the epiphyseal plate. Careful asepsis is essential to reduce the risk of osteomyelitis and I would infiltrate the area down to periosteum with local anaesthetic if the child is conscious. I would direct the needle caudally at 60° to the skin and advance through the cortex with a boring action until I felt a loss of resistance, at which point I should have entered the marrow cavity. I would confirm this by aspirating marrow and then I would carefully secure the needle. The distal tibia proximal to the medial malleolus and the distal femur are alternative sites. Doses of drugs and infusion rates are the same as with the intravenous route, although I would use infusion under pressure for fluid replacement. Once the child's condition improves, I would secure venous access and remove the intraosseous cannula.

The intraosseous route is therefore a safe and highly effective method of obtaining rapid access to the systemic circulation in emergency situations in children under 7 years and in these situations, the procedure may be life-saving.

Q2. OK, what complications of this procedure are known.

Generally speaking, the procedure is safe and in the circumstances when it is used, the benefits far outweigh the risks. However, osteomyelitis is an infrequent but well-recognised complication which occurs in <1% of insertions. Other local complications include cellulitis, abscess formation, compartment syndrome and pain. Fat and bone marrow microemboli are serious but luckily rare systemic complications.

Q3. Fine. Have you ever had to use this procedure?

No, but I have practised the technique on chicken drumsticks in my A&E department. I also know where the intraosseous needles are kept in my hospital.

Tips

- ■ Confidence in emergency medicine is generally difficult to assess in the artificial context of the membership examination so the viva is often chosen by examiners to attempt to test your life-saving skills.

- ■ You will be expected to be familiar with important emergency situations and techniques even if they are uncommon enough to mean that you have no direct experience. One day, they may present in real life and you may not have time to look them up!

REFERENCES

Driggers D A et al 1991 Emergency resuscitation in children. The role of intraosseous infusion. Postgrad Med 89: 129–132

Hapnes S A, Robertson C 1992 CPR-drug delivery routes and systems. A statement for the Advanced Life Support Working Party of the European Resuscitation Council. Resuscitation 24: 137–142

Neonatology

3

Ambiguous genitalia

Q. You are asked to see a baby on the postnatal ward because the baby's sex is not definite. What are you going to do?

Ambiguous genitalia is an uncommon problem, but one that must be dealt with sensitively and appropriately from the start to avoid possible rejection by the family, rearing the infant as the wrong sex and avoiding potential danger to the baby, e.g. salt-losing crisis of congenital adrenal hyperplasia (CAH).

I would inform the parents of the dilemma and explain that the baby should not be named or registered until the correct sex can be determined. I would take immediate action to determine:

1.   *Karyotype.* An urgent result can be obtained within 48 hours of blood being taken.
2.   The presence or absence of a uterus and gonads by *ultrasound scanning of the pelvis.*

From these results one of three broad categories can be differentiated:

a) Male karyotype (XY), palpable gonads, poorly developed male genitalia = *male pseudohermaphroditism*
b) Female karyotype (XX), presence of uterus, masculinisation of external female genitalia = *female pseudohermaphroditism*
c) Mixed karyotype, ambiguous genitalia, both ovarian and testicular tissue = *true hermaphroditism*

Male pseudohermaphroditism — inadequate masculinisation of a male fetus. Although genotypically male, these infants may be best brought up as female, because surgery is more successful at producing a functional vagina than a functional penis. The cause is non-production of testosterone or loss of end-organ responsiveness to the testosterone derivative, dihydrotestosterone.

Causes include:

— gonadal enzyme deficiencies
— gonadal dysgenesis/agenesis
— testicular feminisation: incomplete or complete, i.e. end-organ unresponsiveness

I would initially undertake investigations to determine the level of the block:

— plasma testosterone, dihydrotestosterone
— FSH, LH
— HCG stimulation test (looking for a rise in testosterone levels)
— 17-hydroxyprogesterone

— ± gonadal biopsy

For those with male gonadal tissue, a trial of testosterone can be attempted, looking for a response. If no response occurs (increase in the size of the penis) removal of the tissue is required and the baby should be raised as a girl.

Female hermaphroditism — masculinisation of a female fetus. The vast majority are caused by congenital adrenal hyperplasia, although rarer causes include maternal ingestion of adrogenic drugs and androgen-producing tumours, e.g. arrhenoblastoma, adrenal adenoma.

I would investigate for CAH with serum 17-hydroxyprogesterone, urinary steroid metabolite excretion and for the possibility of salt loss. A salt-losing crisis can occur a number of weeks after delivery and so the baby should not be allowed home until this has been excluded by enzyme estimation and serial serum electrolyte measurement. All thses infants should be raised as female and with appropriate treatment, they may be fertile.

True hermaphroditism. These are usually best reared as female with removal of male gonadal tissue.

A systolic murmur

Q. You hear a systolic murmur in a postnatal check of a baby. What is your management plan?

The answer to this question is dependent on the gestational age of the baby and the clinical status.

As a generality, the vast majority of systolic murmurs heard on the postnatal wards are in well babies who have an innocent murmur. Of those heard on the neonatal ward, the most common is a *patent ductus arteriosus* (PDA) murmur in a premature infant with bounding pulses, active praecordium, etc. However, there are many cardiac causes for a systolic murmur in the newborn, some innocent, some requiring long-term medical follow-up, and others that can be neonatal emergencies.

1. *A murmur in a well term infant on the postnatal ward.*
This is in an infant that is feeding well with no evidence of cyanosis, sweating, pallor, dyspnoea, abnormal or absent pulses, a normal blood pressure, who on auscultation has a short, soft, early systolic murmur, heard only in a small area of the praecordium, with normal heart sounds. This is due either to a flow murmur or a venous hum. I would inform the parents of the findings and arrange follow-up at 6 weeks of age, warning them to bring the infant back sooner if any of the above signs become apparent. If still present then, I would arrange an ECG and chest X-ray, looking for evidence of cardiac pathology. If any abnormality is present, then I would arrange an echocardiogram; otherwise I would simply continue follow-up in the clinic. However, most murmurs will disappear by 6 weeks and the infant can be discharged from the clinic.

2. *An unwell infant with a murmur.*
Only ~1 in 12 murmurs heard in the postnatal period has significant cardiac disease. However, in an unwell infant with a murmur, it must be presumed to be a congenital cardiac lesion until proved otherwise. Any baby who feeds or handles poorly, is sweaty, tachypnoeic, tachycardic, hypotensive or cyanosed, has hepatomegaly or other abnormalities, e.g. cleft lip and palate, or chromosomal syndrome, e.g. Down's syndrome, with a murmur, requires investigation with ECG, chest X-ray and echocardiography. I would transfer the infant to the neonatal unit if not already there, and monitor with ECG and pulse oximetry. The use of the hyperoxic/nitrogen washout test to differentiate between cardiac and respiratory causes of cyanosis is debatable. A PO_2 of >15 kPa (~110 mmHg) after 10 minutes of 100% oxygen administration almost certainly rules out a cardiac cause. However, hyperoxia is a stimulus for closure of the ductus arteriosus, thereby worsening the condition of babies with

duct-dependent cardiac lesions. I would therefore not routinely perform this investigation. Instead, if I presumed a cardiac cause for cyanosis and the infant was unwell, I would start an intravenous prostaglandin infusion, with the intention of re-opening the ductus. I would always ensure adequate ventilation facilities should the infant become apnoeic. Early referral to a specialist paediatric cardiac centre is very important so that detailed ECG studies ± cardiac catheterisations can take place, and if needs be, palliative or corrective surgery.

It is important to bear in mind, that babies with significant congenital cardiac abnormalities may appear extremely well in the first few days of life with no evidence of a murmur. Indeed, the commonest congenital cardiac lesion is a ventricular septal defect and this may not produce a murmur for several weeks.

3. *A murmur on the neonatal unit in a premature infant.*
Naturally a premature infant could have any one of the congenital cardiac abnormalities that a term infant could have. However, the commonest is a PDA. The presence or absence of bounding pulses in a premature infant can be difficult to pick up clinically and babies with a significant PDA may have normal pulses. Colour Doppler ultrasonography is increasingly being used on the neonatal unit. In premature infants with a PDA, I would fluid restrict to around $\frac{2}{3}$ normal. Whether or not I then tried indomethacin (prostaglandin synthetase inhibitor) would depend upon the presence or absence of contraindications (bleeding, intracranial haemorrhage, renal impairment). Ductal ligation under general or local anaesthetic may be necessary.

Jaundice

Q. You are asked to draw up a protocol for the management of jaundiced babies on the postnatal ward. What would you include in this protocol?

The rapid breakdown of fetal haemoglobin and the immaturity of liver-conjugating enzymes result in elevated unconjugated serum bilirubin in neonates. This is physiological jaundice and occurs in up to 50% of term babies and 80% of preterm babies. Not all of these warrant investigation.

In any baby who becomes jaundiced, whether term or preterm, in whom there are concerns, e.g. poor feeding, pale, very jaundiced, dysmorphic, not passing meconium, then a total bilirubin count on heel-prick should be carried out and the paediatrician informed.

Neonates that require further investigation include:

1. Those becoming jaundiced within the first 24 hours, suggesting haemolysis.
2. Marked jaundice or rapidly rising jaundice (>85 mmol/l/day) or jaundice in an unwell baby.
3. Prolonged jaundice beyond 2 weeks of age.

All should have a direct and indirect (conjugated and unconjugated) serum bilirubin and urine check for bilirubin as a minimum.

1. Those becoming *jaundiced in the first 24 hours* usually have haemolysis which may simply be physiological, but could suggest other causes such as ABO or Rhesus incompatibility, red-cell-membrane abnormalities (hereditary spherocytosis, elliptocytosis), red-cell-enzyme deficiencies (glucose-6-phosphate dehydrogenase, pyruvate kinase). Cord blood analysis for Rhesus isoimmunisation should be followed by infant FBC and film, Coomb's test, blood group and SBR. Treatment is dependent upon cause but very often continued monitoring with daily SBRs + phototherapy is the all that is needed. Phototherapy requirements are guided by bilirubin charts.

2. *Marked jaundice or an unwell infant.* Again this marked jaundice may well be physiological, especially if breast fed, but requires investigation as does any unwell infant:

    — full infection screen if unwell
    — thyroid function tests
    — urine culture and reducing substances

Good feeding practice is essential for babies with physiological jaundice. The passage of meconium reduces the enterohepatic circulation of bilirubin. Phototherapy is carried out as necessary.

3. *Prolonged jaundice.* In May 1993 the 'Yellow Alert' National Awareness campaign was launched. Its main purpose was to bring those infants with extra-hepatic biliary atresia (EHBA) to the attention of paediatricians and subsequently paediatric surgeons at an earlier age. Prognosis in EHBA is related to the age at surgery. For those under 2 months, 90% have successful drainage of bile whilst those over 3 months are very unlikely to obtain successful drainage.

Any baby that is still jaundiced requires further investigation — 'split' bilirubin, ALT, urinalysis, stool examination. Conjugated bilirubinaemia (>50 μmol/1) with ALT >50 mmol/1 suggests EBHA.

Many other causes of prolonged and conjugated hyperbilirubinaemia exist and will need exclusion by appropriate investigation.

— α-1 antitrypsin deficiency — α-1 antitrypsin phenotype
— galactosaemia — urine reducing substances and subsequent enzyme assay
— anatomical abnormalities — choledochal cyst, Alagilles' syndrome
— cystic fibrosis — sweat test, immunoreactive trypsin, genetic markers

Retinopathy of prematurity

Q. What is known about the pathogenesis of retinopathy of prematurity?

Retinopathy of prematurity is a *vasoproliferative* disorder which tends to occur in very low birthweight infants. These babies are usually preterm and have immature retinae. The periphery of the retina is incompletely vascularised and therefore susceptible to damage. Any factors which affect the development of the retina may cause retinopathy of prematurity.

Initially it was found that babies who had been exposed to high oxygen levels had a higher risk of retinopathy. This may be due to the formation of *free radicals* which act directly on the immature retina. Careful restriction of oxygen has certainly reduced the incidence of retinopathy, however significant retinopathy still occurs. Retinopathy also occurs in infants who have never had oxygen and those with cyanotic congenital heart disease, suggesting that other factors must be involved.

Vitamin E is an antioxidant thought to protect the retina from oxygen-free radicals. Preterm infants are deficient in vitamin E. Supplementation of vitamin E has not reduced the incidence of retinopathy in those infants studied, although it may have reduced the severity of disease. Little is known about the possible side-effects of vitamin E supplementation and it is not widely used.

Other factors which have been found to be associated with retinoapthy of prematurity include the use of exchange transfusions; recurrent apnoeas; intraventricular haemorrhage and the respiratory distress syndrome. The exact mechanism is not known, but the infants who have these problems are those who are most seriously unwell and therefore more vulnerable to damage. Further research is required to establish pathogenetic factors in order to prevent this disorder.

Hypoglycaemia

Q. When would you consider it necessary to treat neonatal hypoglycaemia?

It is not known what level of blood glucose is physiological for the newborn infant. The neonate has to adjust from a constant glucose supply in utero to an intermittent nutrient supply after birth. In the well term infant, the surge of adrenaline at delivery causes the production of glucagon, cortisol and growth hormone, which allow gluconeogenesis and ketogenesis to proceed. In the first hour after birth, while these adaptations take place, the neonate will have a low blood glucose. This is physiological and does not require correction.

However, a low blood glucose after this initial period is potentially harmful. Traditionally, it has been thought that the preterm infant can tolerate a lower blood glucose then the full term infant. However, recent evidence suggests that persistent glucose levels <2.6 mmol/l may cause permanent neurological damage, especially in small babies. The effects may vary from mild developmental delay to severe cerebral palsy.

A single blood glucose level <2.6 mmol/l in a healthy term infant who is feeding well would not be of great concern, since a well baby can utilise alternative fuel supplies by the production of ketones. However, some infants are at greater risk of hypoglycaemia. Preterm infants are unable to produce ketones and have little subcutaneous tissue to use in gluconeogenesis. Similarly, small for gestational age babies have no substrate to use. Infants who have suffered birth asphyxia have also been found to have reduced ketonic response. Since these infants are often fluid restricted to prevent cerebral oedema, they are at increased risk of hypoglycaemia. Infants of diabetic mothers are prone to hypoglycaemia due to relative hyperinsulinism.

It is important to protect these infants by the introduction of early feeds. In the sicker infants intravenous glucose solutions should be started as soon after delivery as possible. Hypoglycaemia must then be treated vigorously should it occur. It has been shown that persistent moderate hypoglycaemia over a period of days is as potentially damaging as brief profound hypoglycaemia.

Hypoglycaemia can be treated by increasing the amount of glucose supplied to the infant, either intravenously or orally, or by giving glucagon to induce physiological production.

REFERENCES

Hawdon JM, Ward Platt MP, Aynsley-Green A 1994 Prevention and management of neonatal hypoglycaemia. Arch Dis Child 70: F60–65

Mehta, 1994 Prevention and management of neonatal hypoglycaemia. Arch Dis Child 70: F54–65

Extracorporeal membranous oxygenation

Q. What is ECMO and what are its uses in the paediatric population?

Extracorporeal membranous oxygenation is a modified technique of cardiac bypass which allows prolonged *respiratory support* while minimising the *barotrauma* caused by standard mechanical ventilation.

It is performed in specialised centres by draining blood from an artery or vein to a membrane oxygenator, then re-warming the blood before infusing it back via the carotid artery.

It has been used in neonates with good effect when conventional treatment has failed. When careful selection procedures are followed, survival is 80%. Success depends on the primary diagnosis. A national randomised trial is in progress to assess the value of ECMO in the neonatal period.

It can be considered in the following diagnoses:

— meconium aspiration syndrome
— persistent pulmonary hypertension
— congenital diaphragmatic hernia
— respiratory distress syndrome
— pneumonia

The technique is limited to neonates over 35 weeks gestation, who have a birthweight >2 kg due to size of the available cannulation catheters. It is important that end-organ failure, major congenital heart disease and intraventricular haemorrhage are excluded before referral. ECMO is a purely supportive technique used over a period of up to 14 days, allowing oxygenation as the disease process recovers. For this reason it is only of benefit in reversible lung disease. The oxygenation index or alveolar:arterial oxygen difference prior to commencing ECMO may give some indication of predicted mortality.

The hazards of ECMO are mainly technical and are improving as the technique is modified. There is a risk of bleeding problems due to systemic heparinisation, which particularly causes central nervous system haemorrhage. Air embolisation may occur if air is introduced into the circuit. Blood is required to prime the circuit and therefore the risks of blood product exposure need to be considered. The long-term neurological consequences are not yet documented. Ligation of the carotid artery may be important in adult life when further interruption to the circle of Willis would be damaging.

The use of ECMO in the older child is less well assessed due to the smaller numbers involved. However, again it can be used as a rescue technique in severe, but reversible lung disease. It can be considered in the following problems:

— adult respiratory distress syndrome, e.g. following near drowning, smoke inhalation
— viral pneumonia
— respiratory syncitial virus bronchiolitis
— foreign body inhalation
— after major cardiac surgery

This may avoid the effects of barotrauma and be of use where recurrent pneumothoraces are a problem.

ECMO is expensive, but is becoming less invasive and therefore safer. Although at present only used as a last resort, with improvement in the technique it may become useful at an earlier stage in lung disease.

Neonatal fits

Q. You are called to see an infant on the special care baby unit who is having intermittent jerking of all limbs associated with desaturations. How would you manage the infant?

My first priority would be to ensure that the infant has an adequate supply of *oxygen*. I would then quickly consider the most likely cause of a convulsion in this particular child, while arranging for a loading dose of intravenous phenobarbitone to be given if the convulsion continues.

A knowledge of the antenatal and intrapartum history would be important to indicate whether *asphyxia* is a potential problem. A history of prolonged rupture of membranes or maternal pyrexia might suggest a diagnosis of *meningitis*. It would be useful to know whether the mother had been using any drugs during her pregnancy which might cause a *withdrawal reaction* in an infant of a few days old.

Metabolic disturbances are a common cause of convulsions in the neonatal period and should be excluded promptly since correction of the primary abnormality will stop the convulsion. I would take blood to check glucose, calcium, sodium and magnesium levels. Blood cultures, full blood count and screening for congenital infections should also be done.

In most cases the convulsion will stop after a loading dose of phenobarbitone. However, if the fit continues, I would give a loading dose of phenytoin slowly while monitoring the cardiac rhythm. Rarely, the convulsion continues and I would then start a clonazepam infusion. This is usually very effective, but of course has a sedative effect, which in combination with the other medications may depress respiratory effort profoundly. In this situation the infant will need ventilation.

Once the convulsion has been controlled, I would continue investigating the cause. If the infant is too unstable to endure a lumbar puncture and no definite cause has been established for the fit, I would start high-dose broad-spectrum antibiotics until meningitis can be excluded. I would arrange a cranial ultrasound, which may show subdural or, less commonly, intraventricular haemorrhage. Rarely, structural abnormalities of the brain, such as lissencephaly, may present with neonatal seizures.

A strong *family history* of fits in the early neonatal period, which subsequently resolved, might be reassuring. Seizures which occur on the second or third day of life, when the infant is well interictally, may be accounted for by a familial trait and are usually self-limiting.

The duration of anticonvulsant treatment will depend on the cause of the convulsion. Once the convulsions have ceased, I would withdraw one drug at a time over a period of several days. Long-term maintenance anticonvulsants will sometimes be required if convulsions recur.

It is important to discuss the implications of the convulsion with the parents. I would explain that the prognosis is unpredictable, but it is reassuring if the convulsion was brief or due to a transient metabolic disturbance. The clinical state of the infant will also affect outcome. An infant who has retained normal tone and activity postictally may have a better prognosis than one that remains flaccid. I would strongly recommend immunising the baby against pertussis, particularly if the fits were transient and the cause is identified.

Breastfeeding

Q1. Tell me about breastfeeding.

The bottom line is that breastfeeding is the overall ideal method of infant nutrition and should be strongly encouraged.

The advantages to the *baby* are:

1. An overall lower infant mortality rate.
2. Protection against infection by conveying IgA, lysozyme, lymphocytes (containing interferon) and macrophages, therefore transmitting both humoral and cellular immunity.
3. Breast milk is acid therefore promoting the growth of 'friendly' lactobacillus in the baby's bowel.
4. Breast milk contains lactoferrin, an iron-binding protein, which inhibits pathogenic *E. coli* and also promotes growth of lactobacilli. Gastroenteritis is therefore reduced by these two mechanisms as well as by the immune ones.
5. Breast milk contains less sodium, potassium and chloride than other milks, thus reducing the risk of fatal hypernatraemia in states of dehydration.
6. In the first 2 or 3 days after birth, colostrum rather than milk is produced. This is yellower and more watery than milk (in fact some primiparous mothers believe their milk is 'bad' and therefore need reassurance). Colostrum is especially rich in IgA and contains some IgM and is important in conferring early 'first-line' defences to the baby's GI tract. IgA protects from both viral and bacterial infection.
7. The protein in breast milk is less likely to induce allergic reactions and this may, in part, protect against sudden infant death.
8. Babies born to atopic parents show a reduced tendency to eczema if they are breastfed.
9. Breast milk contains substances such as taurine and long-chain fatty acids that are important in development. Some studies have actually suggested that breastfed infants attain a higher IQ than those who are bottle-fed.
10. Breastfeeding is a natural way of promoting bonding between mother and baby.
11. It is more interesting for the baby as the maternal diet changes the taste!

The advantages to the *mother* are:

1. Breastfeeding is cheap, easy, convenient and clean. It is supplied pre-prepared, pre-heated and sterile!

2. It is a 'total experience', stimulating all five senses and aiding the bonding process.
3. Suckling promotes uterine contraction therefore reducing the risk of postpartum haemorrhage.
4. Full breastfeeding provides reasonable contraception due to the suppression of ovulation by prolactin.
5. Carcinoma of the breast is less common in women who have breastfed.

Despite these numerous advantages over bottle feeding, the proportion of women who breastfeed has declined since the late 1970s and remains low throughout Britain (Emery et al 1990). The Office of Population Censuses and Surveys suggests a national prevalence of breastfeeding of only 41% at 7 days in 1990 and Howie et al (1990) showed that the prevalence is lower in socially deprived areas.

Q2. What do you know about the constituents of breast milk?

Breast milk contains about 70 kcal of energy per 100 ml compared to 66 kcal in cow's milk and 65 kcal in formula milk. There is considerably less protein in breast milk (1.0 g/dl compared to 1.8 g/dl for formula milk and 3.5 g/dl for cow's milk). Breast milk protein is composed largely of whey which contains lactalbumin as well as lactoferrin and the immune proteins. Whey is more digestible than casein which is the major cow's milk protein. Casein is more likely to precipitate in the stomach as curd which, though important in the regulation of stomach emptying, can lead to curd obstruction.

Breast milk contains a greater proportion of essential polyunsaturated fatty acids and cholesterol than cow's or formula milk. Lipase enzyme is present in breast milk only and is responsible for liberating fatty acids which are important sources of energy for the baby.

Almost all the carbohydrate in the three types of milk is lactose and the amount in breast milk is considerably more than in cow's milk (7.5 g/dl compared to 5 g/dl) but about the same as in formula (7 g/dl). Lactose is easily metabolised to galactose which is vital for normal myelin formation and brain development. It is also fermented by gut lactobacilli to produce an acid stool.

Breast milk has higher levels of vitamins A, C and E than cow's milk, though less vitamin K, which may predispose to haemorrhagic disease of the newborn. The Department of Health recommends that vitamin drops are given to all breastfed babies.

I have already mentioned colostrum which is produced in the first couple of days and is rather thin and watery and has a lower fat and carbohydrate content compared to milk. It is, however, rich in protein. Constituents also change during a feed with milk at the end of a feed, hind milk, being richer in fat than fore milk.

Q3. You've mentioned the numerous advantages of breast milk. Why do you think many mothers don't breastfeed?

When I have asked mothers on postnatal wards why they have chosen not to breastfeed, I have encountered a variety of reasons. Some women just do not like the idea of breastfeeding and family or peer-related attitudes are probably very relevant here. Others lack self-confidence, are embarrassed or fear that they will develop painful, swollen breasts. Several women begin breastfeeding but give up because they believe, wrongly, that they are producing inadequate amounts of milk and are not satisfying their baby.

Many women are also under the mistaken impression that bottle feeding is easier and less disruptive. In virtually all circumstances, this is the opposite of the truth. Once established, breastfeeding is very convenient and though not perfect, there is now reasonable provision of nursing rooms in public places.

In many of these cases, I believe that adequate and sympathetic *health education*, both antenatally and on a continuing basis by the GP, midwife, obstetrician, paediatrician and health visitor, would improve the understanding and acceptance of breastfeeding. School and media education also has an important role.

Q4. OK, what are the contraindications to breastfeeding?

These are relatively few. Maternal ones are certain drugs, severe ill-health and being hepatitis B HBsAg positive. Maternal HIV carriage is a contentious issue. It has generally been regarded as a contraindication though many authorities believe that if the baby has escaped infection in utero, the benefits may outweigh the small added risk.

Neonatal ones are anatomical abnormalities of the mouth such as cleft palate and certain inherited metabolic diseases such as PKU, galactosaemia and mono- and disaccharide intolerances.

Tips

■ Note how easy it is to 'pull yourself' into the answer (". .I have asked mothers on postnatal wards. ."), which gives you the air of experience and enthusiasm and also adds flavour to your response. Make your answers stand out from the hundreds the examiners have already endured that day.

■ This type of question gives you good ground on which to demonstrate that you have a wider understanding of health issues such as health education and social awareness.

REFEFENCES

Emery J L et al 1990 Decline in breast-feeding. Arch Dis Child 65: 369–372
Howie P W et al 1990 Protective effects of breast-feeding against infection. Br Med J 300: 11–16

Steroids

Q. What do you consider to be the role of corticosteroids on the neonatal unit?

Corticosteroids have a role in both the prevention and treatment of lung disease in the preterm infant.

They have been shown to be useful in the prevention of *respiratory distress syndrome*, reducing incidence by as much as 50%, if given to the mother prior to delivery. They act by stimulating surfactant synthesis in the alveolar type II cells. They also seem to accelerate maturation of the fetal lung. Dexamethasone is most frequently used since it is the steroid that is least inactivated by the placenta.

The side-effects of steroids on the fetus need to be considered. If large doses are given there may be suppression of the fetal adrenal glands causing low endogenous cortisol synthesis. In practice, this is not a problem at currently used doses.

If steroids are given too early before delivery, fetal growth may be affected. The maximum benefit is probably achieved when given 48 hours before delivery in a threatened preterm labour. The gestation at which steroids should be used is not certain, however they are of proven benefit in mothers <30 weeks and I would consider their use in those <34 weeks. I would avoid giving steroids to mothers who have had prolonged rupture of membranes or signs of developing infection.

Intravenous or oral dexamethasone may also be used in the preterm infant with *chronic lung disease*. Infants who are still ventilated or in high quantities of oxygen at 3 weeks may benefit from a course of steroids. It has been shown that steroids reduce the length of time ventilated or oxygen dependent in these infants. A long but reducing course of dexamethasone has been generally most effective in the management of chronic lung disease.

In the short term the toxic effects of steroids include:

— hypertension
— hyperglycaemia and consequent glycosuria
— susceptibility to infection, particularly fungal infection
— poor growth

All infants on a course of steroids should be closely observed for these problems. Less well known are the long-term effects on the infant, e.g. on the development of the infant brain. For this reason, I would give careful consideration before prescribing a course of dexamethasone.

There has been recent interest in the use of inhaled steroids in the oxygen-dependant neonate. These are effectively a topical treatment and therefore may reduce the incidence of side-effects.

Finally, I have found a short course of corticosteroids to be useful in the management of the ventilated infant with laryngeal oedema, who develops marked stridor and fatigue on extubation.

Surfactant

Q1. What is surfactant and what role does it have in neonatology?

Surfactant is a natural substance produced in utero by the developing lungs from around the 24th week by alveolar type 2 cells, secreted by and stored in lamellar bodies. It has a complex make up consisting primarily of phospholipids and protein (SPA-A, SPA-B, SPA-C and SPA-D). The phospholipid phosphatidylcholine is the main component of surfactant enabling it to form a monolayer over the alveolar surface. This has two major effects:

1. Lowers the surface tension of the alveoli and so reduces the work of expansion
2. Prevents atelectasis

Deficiency of surfactant is synonymous with respiratory distress syndrome (RDS) in preterm infants, but it is important to realise that there is more to RDS than straightforward surfactant deficiency.

There are several types of surfactant on the market:

— Curosurf : porcine derived
— Exosurf (coloscent palmitate) : synthetic
— ALEC (Artificial Lung Expanding Compound) : synthetic
— Survanta : cow/calf derived

All have been the subject of extensive research and the majority of the trials suggest an overall reduction in mortality of around 40%, but generally no reduction in morbidity (periventricular haemorrhage, intraventricular haemorrhage, bronchopulmonary dysplasia), apart from pneumothorax. The largest and best known trial was OSIRIS (Open Study of Infants at high risk or with Respiratory Insufficiency — the role of Surfactant) coordinated by the National Perinatal Epidemiology Unit in Oxford. This trial looked at the administration of Exosurf, particularly early *vs* rescue administration and dosage frequency. Their main conclusions were:

1. There is no clear difference in mortality between early and rescue administration.
2. There is a reduction in the risk of pneumothorax with early administration.
3. There is no additional benefit of continued administration after the standard two doses 12 hours apart.
4. There is unnecessary extra use of surfactant in 25% of babies randomised to early treatment.

There is no doubt that in the future, the administration of surfactant to preterm infants will be incorporated into standard treatment management, but it is at present a very expensive treatment and requires careful studies, research and audit.

Q2. What other treatment options are there for RDS?

1. *Antenatal administration of steroids.*
This is a very cheap and effective way of increasing endogenous surfactant production within the lungs of preterm infants. Trials suggest that administration should take place at least 6 hours prior to delivery and ideally for a period of 48 hours between 1 and 7 days before delivery. Most hospitals give antenatal steroids to eligible mothers only if the gestation is <34 weeks — above this age, mortality from RDS is very low.

The mechanism of action of antenatal steroids has not been fully elucidated. However, it is known that steroids act on lung fibroblasts to induce production of fibroblast pneumocyte factor. This has a positive effect on the alveolar type 2 cell production of surfactant. Steroids may also aid development of adrenergic receptors on alveolar type 2 cells in utero, increasing surfactant production at the time of the adrenergic surge of delivery.

2. *Antenatal administration of thyrotrophin releasing hormone.*
Used in combination with steroids, this appears to have an additive effect upon surfactant release.

REFERENCES

Berger H M et al 1994 The in's and out's of RDS in babies and adults. J R Coll Physicians Lond 28: 24–33
Morley C J 1992 Surfactant. In: Roberton NRC (ed) Textbook of neonatology. Churchill Livingstone, Edinburgh, Ch 11
Morley C J 1991 Surfactant treatment of premature infants. Arch Dis Child 66: 445–504
The OSIRIS Collaborative group 1992 Early versus delayed neonatal administration of a synthetic surfactant — the judgement of OSIRIS. Lancet 340: 1363–1369
Wilkinson A R 1993 Surfactant therapy In: David T (ed) Recent Advances in Paediatrics 11: 53–66

Antenatal screening

Q. What antenatal screening takes place in the UK?

Ideally all women who are thinking of having a baby should, prior to conceiving, attend the GP for general advice. At this appointment the GP can advice regarding smoking, alcohol consumption, coming off contraception, diet, maintaining good glycaemic control for patients with diabetes, avoidance of drugs or modification of drug therapies to prevent harm to the developing fetus, vitamin and folate supplementation. Whether this can be considered screening is debatable, and although very important, I wonder how frequently it happens in reality.

Screening usually starts when a prospective mother first attends the GP to confirm the pregnancy (usually when the second period has been missed). Every mother should have blood taken for haemoglobin, blood group, rubella status, syphilis serology and hepatitis serology. As well as full history and examination, an assessment of risk for the pregnancy is made. For those with high risk, e.g. poor obstetric history, older mothers, complex medical problems, early referral to the hospital obstetricians is advised. For the less 'at risk' pregnancy, the standard procedure is shared care between GP and hospital with antenatal visits every 6–8 weeks until 28 weeks, then fortnightly until 36 weeks and thereafter weekly until delivery. At these visits, mothers are weighed, blood pressure is recorded, urine is tested for protein and glucose and fundal height and lie palpated. Listening for the fetal heart is also undertaken.

All pregnant women should have a booking in ultrasound scan of the fetus and placenta. The detail obtained by ultrasound scan is becoming very good indeed. General measurements carried out are biparietal diameter, abdominal trunk diameter and trunk area. The condition of the placenta and volume of amniotic fluid are also assessed. Anatomy of the baby can be looked at and nowadays minor details can be observed, which are not harmful to the baby, but potentially shocking to the parents if not forewarned, e.g. absent toes, cleft lip. More life-threatening abnormalities can also be picked up, e.g. spina bifida, hydrops fetalis, encephalocoele. Identifying minor abnormalities may or may not be productive. On the one hand forewarned is forarmed, but on the other the knowledge may create anxiety, often out of proportion to the degree of abnormality.

Other screening tests include:

1. *The triple test.*
Used for the diagnosis of Down's syndrome. Prior to its introduction, screening for Down's involved the offer of amniocentesis to those women over a certain age, e.g. 35. However, this screening was not particularly successful as most

Down's babies are born to women under 35 years, and uptake of amniocentesis was not 100%. The triple test, together with maternal age, is a better predictor of risk and allows more specific directions for offering diagnostic amniocentesis. It involves taking a sample of blood between 15 and 20 weeks of pregnancy and measuring serum α-fetoprotein, unconjugated oestriol and human chorionic gonodotrophin. A risk score is calculated and all those with a score of 1 in 250 or less are offered an amniocentesis. Correct assessment of gestational age is imperative for the results to be valid. Prior to the introduction of the triple test around 900 babies a year were born with Down's syndrome. Some estimates put the rate with current screening as low as 300 a year but this may not be accurate.

2. *Daily fetal movement count.*
From 9 am the time is recorded for 10 fetal movements to occur. If these do not occur within 12 hours on consecutive days, the woman should report to the hospital.

3. *Cytogenetic screening.*
This is not yet standard practice, but there are many genetic disorders for which screening is available. By means of chorionic villous sampling (CVS) or amniocentesis, fetal cells are obtained and cytogenetics and DNA analyses can be carried out. These invasive prodedures with their attendant risks (procedure related loss = 1–2% for amniocentesis, 2–3% for CVS) are offered to those mothers in whom potential gains outweigh risk.

4. *HIV screening.*
In some health authorities in the UK, pregnant mothers are screened anonymously at booking for HIV infection. This conveys no advantage to the women or her baby, but provides very useful epidemiological information.

5. *New concepts.*
Looking to the future, I have recently read about a very interesting technique for antenatal diagnosis. Fetal blood cells can be found and isolated from a maternal blood sample whilst pregnant due to the presence of fetal haemoglobin. If a PCR technique could be applied to the fetal cells, then theoretically enough genetic material could be obtained to perform cytogenetic analysis on the amplified fetal DNA, thus negating the need for invasive sampling techniques.

REFERENCES

Wald N J et al 1988 Maternal serum screening for Down's syndrome in early pregnancy. Br Med J 297: 883–887

Wald N J et al 1992 Antenatal maternal serum screening for Down's syndrome. Results of a demonstration project. Br Med J 305: 391–396

Hypoxic ischaemic encephalopathy

Q. What do you understand by hypoxic ischaemic encephalopathy (HIE)?

HIE is a clinical neurological syndrome ocurring in neonates and is related to prenatal, natal and postnatal *asphyxia*. Anaerobic metabolism resulting in accumulation of lactate produces acidosis and disruption of lysosome function. Cerebral oedema develops and, together with hypotension, cerebral perfusion pressure falls and ischaemia ensues.

HIE can be divided into three grades:

— *Grade 1:* poor sucking, mild hypotonia, hyperalertness
— *Grade 2:* lethargy, absent suck, hypotonia, convulsions very common
— *Grade 3:* stuporous/comatose, flaccid tone, prolonged fits, absent sucking and Moro reflexes, requiring ventilatory support. Intracranial pressure (ICP) is elevated

Diagnosis is essentially clinical, supported by cerebral function monitoring, measurement of intracranial pressure and radiological investigation as available.

Management ideally would be prediction of those infants at risk of HIE and appropriate intervention to prevent cerebral ischaemia. For infants presumed to have suffered an hypoxic ischaemic episode around the time of delivery, suggested by poor Apgar scores, close observation is necessary. Correction of derangements of temperature and serum glucose, coupled with apnoea and transcutaneous O_2/CO_2 monitoring must be carried out. Blood gas analysis to prevent hypoxaemia/hyperoxaemia and hypercapnia should be undertaken every 4 hours at least. Blood pressure measurement and maintenance is essential to prevent less than optimal cerebral perfusion. In all but mild HIE, fits are common, although sometimes difficult to detect. Hypoglycaemia and hypocalcaemia must be corrected and fits treated aggressively. First-line treatment is phenobarbitone, a loading dose, followed by continuous i.v. infusion. If unsuccessful, other anticonvulsants may be used, e.g. paraldehyde, diazepam.

The control of raised ICP is contentious and possibly of limited benefit. Current thinking is to try and minimise cerebral oedema by fluid restriction to $\frac{2}{3}$ of maintenance and hyperventilation. Possible manoeuvres for the future may include glutamate receptor blockers, calcium channel blockers and free radical inhibitors.

Asphyxial damage to other organs of the body will need consideration and possible treatment, e.g. acute renal failure, DIC, septicaemia.

Finally, discussion with the parents is important. Prognosis is difficult to predict, but those infants with evidence of significant asphyxia, i.e. profound acidosis on fetal scalp pH sampling, low Apgar scores, convulsions, etc. must have a guarded outcome. Generally, those with grade 1 HIE have no neurological sequelae and those with grade 3 have severe neurological deficit if they survive.

Ethical dilemmas on the neonatal unit

Q. What are your views on the ethics of neonatal medicine?

In no other speciality of medicine are there more ethical dilemmas than in neonatology. Every day the neonatologist is faced with the decision shall I or shall I not treat? No two situations are the same and no two neonatologists would always agree on the same situation. Very often the decision to continue or not (or indeed start) is in the hands of the most junior doctor who is present 24 hours a day on the baby unit. Guidelines can be drawn up, but ultimately the decision is made by the attending doctor and provided that it is made in the patient's best interest, then the doctor should receive the support of his/her colleagues.

The problem then is what constitutes the patient's interests — the patient is not able to describe these interests and their voice must be through the parents. Three general situations exists.

1.   An infant born with an anencephaly will not survive and virtually all of us would accept that *selective non-treatment* is in the patient's interests. The difficulty arises if the parents feel that there is hope and that everything should be done to try and salvage the baby. If a fatal outcome is expected from prenatal investigation, the consultant paediatrician in charge should sit down with the parents and family and explain the likely prognosis. In this way, the views of the parents can be expressed prior to delivery and before the need for difficult decisions arises. If the weight of medical opinion is laid down on the table, almost certainly the parents will allow the doctors to make the critical decisions at delivery. It is essential to avoid confusing or contradictory advice from a host of different sources.

This is an ideal situation and one that rarely happens. More often there is no warning, e.g. a mother comes into hospital as an emergency in late labour, pushing at 23 weeks, and the baby delivers as the paediatrician arrives. A brief history at the time may give confusion over dates and gestation and so the paediatrician is faced with a difficult decision. A baby of <500g with fused eyelids, gelatinous skin, etc. is extremely unlikely to survive in the first instance and even if survival is possible, severe handicap may almost be inevitable. In that situation my feelings would be a very limited resuscitation initially (suction, face mask oxygen + bag and mask). If there is no dramatic improvement, I would not continue, as once intensive treatment has been initiated, pulling out from this is very hard (although some would consider that there is no difference between withholding and withdrawing treatment). Once a baby has been intubated and ventilated, I would continue intensive treatment until such time that the situation appears hopeless (e.g. grade IV IVH, profound, prolonged acidosis).

The time to *withdraw* occurs after full and open discussion with the parents and nursing staff. If parents still feel that everything should be done, the decision may then have to be taken away from them. To expend limited resources on an infant who in the medical opinion will die anyway, must be morally wrong (and legally wrong, as the Court of Appeal has judged).

2. The converse to the situation is the *parent who wants nothing done*, but the doctor feels that something must be done, e.g. an infant of a diabetic mother who is hypoglycaemic and not feeding but the mother is refusing nasogastric feeds, glucagon or i.v. glucose therapy. The doctor has every right to administer these therapies against the parents' wishes to save the babies life.

3. The third intermediate situation is the baby whose *outcome cannot be predicted* with any degree of certainty. Benefit of the doubt must be given and treatment carried out, until such time that it becomes clear what the outcome will be.

In conclusion, there can be no rules for the ethical issues highlighted above. Each situation has to be judged at the time for the best interest of the patient. Decisions made should always be in association with the parents and family unless medical guidelines dictate otherwise. Accurate documentation of discussions and decisions must always be made in the medical records.

Breaking bad news

Q. How would you break bad news to a family on the neonatal unit?

Ideally, the most experienced person available should break any bad news to the family. However, if a direct question is asked, it is important that the family do not feel they are being avoided. I would want to speak to both parents together and include another family member or friend if they wish. I would see the parents in a private area, with the baby nearby if possible. Tissues should be within easy reach.

A nurse or health visitor, who may know the family well, should be present. This allows the family to talk about the nature of the news with someone professional after the interview is complete. I would aim to be sympathetic and gentle in my approach, while telling the news in a factual manner using uncomplicated language.

The family may be aware that the baby is seriously unwell and may have prepared questions to ask. It is essential to listen carefully to the parents and not to interrupt. The shock of the news may be taken calmly initially, however the family may react with grief or anger. The natural instinct is to comfort the family and this is an appropriate reaction which may be met with gratitude. It does no harm for the parents to see our own emotional reaction and physical contact may be appreciated.

It is easy to give the parents a lot of information at this interview, but much will be forgotten and a further meeting should be arranged. I would write a summary of what has been said in the notes so that all staff can be aware of the discussion should further explanations be required.

When talking to the parents of a child with a visible abnormality which is not necessarily fatal, such as a baby with Down's syndrome or a cleft palate, I feel that it is helpful to demonstrate the abnormalities one by one, rather than showing them the problems all at once. This allows them to adapt slowly. If an operation is likely, 'before and after' photographs can be shown. Literature relevant to the disorder and information about support groups should be given, if available. Parents naturally have high expectations of their newborn baby and any abnormality, however minor it seems to us, is of great significance to the family. Care must be taken to treat any such problems as 'bad news'.

Cardiology and respiratory medicine

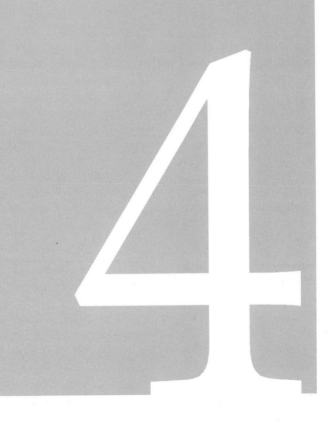

4

Endocarditis

Q1. Tell me about the clinical features of bacterial endocarditis.

The division into acute and subacute bacterial endocarditis is generally no longer made microbiologically, although it is clinically important to be aware that the disease may present in both a rather indolent non-specific fashion or with a florid fulminant picture. In children, *congenital heart disease* (CHD) rather than rheumatic fever is the usual predisposing problem, although this may not have been previously diagnosed. Recent studies have shown an almost equal incidence in cyanotic and acyanotic CHD.

The classic triad of the clinical features of endocarditis should now be considered as a tetrad.

— infection
— heart disease
— embolism
— immunological disease

1. *Features of infection.*
These include *fever*, possibly with drenching night sweats and rigors, lassitude, arthralgia and myalgia. *Splenomegaly* is present in at least two-thirds of cases. Failure to thrive and anaemia may be prominent in more indolent cases.

It is important to remember that in subacute presentations, fever may be mild or in rare cases even absent and the child may merely present with apathy and vague ill-health.

2. *Features of heart disease.*
In the majority of conditions, careful examination of the heart will reveal signs of any pre-existing valvular or shunt-related disease with or without signs of the endocarditis. Any *murmur* in the face of an unexplained pyrexial illness should alert the clinician to the possibility of endocarditis. The blowing early-diastolic murmur of aortic regurgitation and the loud pansystolic murmur of mitral regurgitation should especially be sought as these are frequent complicating lesions. These arise because of the destruction of valve leaflets by the infected vegetations. Any murmur which has changed from a previous examination should especially arouse suspicion.

Finger clubbing may develop in subacute disease or may have already been present in cases of congenital cyanotic heart disease. Hepatomegaly, with or without palpable pulsation and other signs of heart failure, may be present.

3. *Features of embolism.*

Any child with unexpected embolism should be suspected as having endocarditis and this is now an important cause of death in this illness. The risk of septic embolism and the subsequent development of mycotic aneurysm (here this term implies infective rather than fungal!) is substantially reduced by early diagnosis and treatment.

The brain, kidneys, liver, spleen and bone are particular sites for emboli (with predictable consequences) and therefore also for the development of secondary foci of infection.

4. *Features of immunological disease.*

Many of the 'classic' signs of endocarditis which were previously thought to be embolic are now known to represent immunological phenomena. The mechanism of these features is thought to be antigen–antibody–complement complexes being deposited in tissues.

These features are of particular importance as, though subtle, they may precede the more severe manifestations. Their early recognition may therefore be life-saving. They are:

a) *Splinter haemorrhages* which are linear subungual haemorrhages present on fingers and occasionally on toes. They are distinguishable from traumatic splinter haemorrhages on the basis that their distal end does not reach the distal end of the nail bed.

b) *Petechial lesions* in endocarditis characteristically have a pale centre and tend to be found on the conjunctivae, dorsum of the hands, oral mucous membranes and the trunk.

c) *Osler's nodes* are relatively uncommon in children. They are painful small red/purple raised lesions found on the pulp of the terminal phalanges of the fingers.

d) *Janeway lesions* are flat, non-tender, erythematous lesions found on the thenar or hypothenar eminences.

e) *Roth's spots* are white-centred haemorrhages found on the retina. A careful search for these should be made, if necessary after dilation of the pupil, in any child seriously suspected as having endocarditis.

f) A *diffuse glomerulonephritis* with changes which may be identical to those found in proliferative glomerulonephritis is often found. This will cause microscopic haematuria which should always be looked for by urine microscopy (rather than just dip-sticking the urine).

Because endocarditis is not frequently encountered in paediatrics, it may be easily missed in the early stages unless the condition is specifically considered and the manifestations carefully sought. Compounding this is the fact that the features of endocarditis, particularly in the early stages, may be very subtle. Recognising a changing heart murmur or the various immunological phenomena in a restless infant requires special clinical skills. Additionally, the child may present with a very atypical picture such as pulmonary infarction, or apparently 'pure' nephritis or heart failure (Channer et al 1989). Early recognition and prompt treatment (usually blind) is vital to minimise the considerable mortality and morbidity associated with this condition.

Tip

■ You may never have seen a case of childhood endocarditis but, because of its nature, the examiner will expect you to demonstrate some knowledge of its possible clinical manifestations.

REFERENCE

Channer K S et al 1989 Presentation of infective endocarditis in childhood and adolescence. J R Col Physicians 23: 152–155

Complications of congenital heart disease

Q1. What complications of congenital heart disease are you aware of?

Congenital heart disease occurs in the UK with an incidence of 8 per 1000 live births. Eight specific abnormalities account for at least 80% of these, namely VSD, PDA, ASD, tetralogy of Fallot, pulmonary stenosis, coarctation, aortic stenosis and transposition of the great arteries. Only 25–30% of cases are recognised in the first year of life; a significant proportion of these presenting in the neonatal period with either cyanosis (TGA, pulmonary atresia/stenosis, tricuspid atresia, Ebstein's anomaly) or heart failure (hypoplastic left heart syndrome, coarctation, severe aortic stenosis). Less dramatically, a baby can be picked up simply by the presence of a murmur and subsequent investigation.

Prompt recognition and appropriate treatment is essential for survival and maximal growth and development potential for every child.

Complications of congenital heart disease can be divided usefully into three groups:

1. Short-term complications
2. Long-term complications
3. Risk of recurrence in siblings and offspring

1. *Short-term complications*
Briefly alluded to above, heart failure and cyanosis can be the presentation of underlying heart disease, but are really considered a consequence rather than complication. They require immediate attention to prevent or minimise insult to the brain, heart, lungs, liver and kidneys. Specific treatment is dependent upon the most likely diagnosis, but would include prostaglandin E1 for duct-dependent lesions, assisted ventilation and inotropic support, as well as correction of hypoxia, acidosis and hypoglycaemia.

2. *Long-term complications*
a) *Growth and development*. Long-term follow up studies of children with congenital heart disease have shown that the uncomplicated acyanotic obstructive lesions have a normal growth pattern without developmental delay. However, those with shunting of blood both from left to right and right to left sides of the heart show an affected growth pattern with weight and height delay proportional to the size of the shunt. Delay in acquisition

of motor skills has been documented in those with shunts and those with right to left shunts have shown a significant lowering of IQ.

b) *Thrombosis and embolism*. Cerebral vessel thrombosis is fortunately rare but a potentially disastrous complication of congenital heart disease. Polycythaemia and a raised haematocrit produce an increased coaguable state, exacerbated by dehydration. Therefore, gastroenteritis, pyrexias, poor feeding, etc., which can lead to dehydration, should have a lower threshold for treatment than for a 'normal' child.

   Paradoxical embolisation following the breaking off a mural thrombus from within the heart in cyanotic congenital heart disease and cerebral abscess formation are again potentially life threatening, though rare complications.

c) *Infective endocarditis*. This is an uncommon complication especially in those under 24 months. It is associated with dental surgery in only a minority of cases. Notoriously difficult to diagnose, it requires thought in any child with congenital heart disease and a pyrexia of unknown origin. Serial blood cultures and detailed echocardiography aid diagnosis.

d) *Cardiac arrhythmia*. Supraventricular tachycardia occurs most frequently in children with a structurally normal heart, but classically occurs in adults with atrial septal defects and in Ebstein's anomaly. Cardiac surgery can result in disruption or damage to the conducting system of the heart, requiring medical or further surgical intervention.

e) *Pulmonary hypertension*. This has been divided into three groups:
   — passive pulmonary hypertension from the transmission of back pressure from the left side of the heart to the pulmonary vasculature
   — hyperdynamic pulmonary hypertension because of the increased blood flow through the pulmonary vasculature
   — reactive pulmonary hypertension from pulmonary artery constriction secondary to local hypoxia

   If pulmonary hypertension is severe and prolonged, Eisenmenger's syndrome can arise resulting in reversed or bidirectional blood flow across the heart. Heart–lung transplantation is the only treatment available once this situation is reached.

f) *Sudden death*. The association with hypertrophic obstructive cardiomyopathy is well known but in any left-sided obstructive lesions, cardiac output tends to fall with exercise. Therefore, constraints must be placed upon those people. Unoperated cyanotic congenital heart disease patients should also avoid recreational exercise.

g) *Miscellaneous*.

— travel: this creates two problems. Those with congestive heart failure, cyanotic heart disease or pulmonary hypertension can fly but should travel with supplemental oxygen during the flight to reduce the risk of thrombosis formation. Holiday destinations with a warm climate can result in increased sweating and the risk of dehydration and thrombosis formation.

— career ambitions: declaration of one's medical history may prejudice against desired employment.

— pregnancy: this can place an unacceptable increased demand on the heart and so any woman contemplating starting a family who has congenital heart disease should seek appropriate advice prior to conceiving. It must also be born in mind that the oral contraceptive pill and the intrauterine contraceptive device may be contraindicated in certain conditions, e.g. pulmonary hypertension, prosthetic heart valves and cyanotic congenital heart disease.

— acquisition of life insurance. This may prove impossible or prohibitively expensive for those with congential heart disease. In the majority this will be unfair discrimination, but Brackenridge guidelines exist as a means of assessing increased risk of death.

3. *Risk of recurrence*

Most congenital heart defects are presumed to have a multifactorial inheritance pattern. The risk of a couple having a second child with congenital heart disease is put between 1 and 5%. Because children with congenital heart disease are now surviving to adulthood and reproductibility, they are passing on an increased risk to their offspring. The figures quoted for the size of this risk varies significantly and some have put it as high as 15%. Only further long-term studies will be able to assess this risk more accurately.

Q2. You have mentioned infective endocarditis as a complication of congenital heart disease. What recommendations would you give for antibiotic cover for such a child?

In all, good oral hygeine and regular dental check-ups are imperative. The family should be made aware of the need for antibiotic cover for certain procedures so that this information can be passed onto the attending physician/dentist.

1. For dental surgery:

— 3 g oral amoxycillin 1 hour before the procedure
— 1.5 g in under 10 year olds
— erythromycin 1 g 1 hour before for those with sensivity to penicillins

2. Gastrointestinal and genitourinary surgery:

— 2 mg/kg i.m. gentamicin + 1 g i.m. ampicillin

3. Prosthetic valves:
   — 1 g i.m. ampicillin 1 g i.m. cloxacillin 1 hour before and doses 8 and
     16 hours after the procedure

REFERENCES

Brackenridge RDC 1985 Medical selection of life risks: a comprehensive guide to life expertancy for underwriters and clinicians. Macmillan, London, pp. 241–261

Suoninen p 1971 Physical growth of children with congenital heart disease: Pre and post operative study of 335 cases. Acta Paed Scand (Suppl) 225: 1–45

Kawasaki disease

Q. Tell me about the interesting condition of Kawasaki disease.

Kawasaki disease/acute febrile muco-cutaneous lymph node syndrome is now the commonest recognised cause of acquired heart disease in childhood. The condition was first monitored in the UK by a joint BPA/CDSC venture in 1983, but from 1986 to 1993 it was under the BPSU surveillance. Their results suggest an increased incidence or increased awareness of the disease until the 1990s, since when numbers seem to have levelled off at about 170 cases a year (3–4 cases per 100 000 < 5 year olds in the UK in 1990, compared with 172 cases per 100 000 <5 year olds in 1986 in Japan). Male to female ratio is about 2:1 and 75% of cases occur in the under 5 year age group.

Aetiology is uncertain — evidence of person-to-person transmission is not substantive, but an infectious cause is an attractive one. Several associations have been postulated such as carpet shampoo, house dust mite, *Proprionobacterium acnes* and retroviruses, but none of these has been proven.

The underlying pathological process is a diffuse vasculitis affecting small and medium sized blood vessels. Demonstrable acute T and B cell changes have been found, which may explain the efficacy of immunoglobulins in some studies.

Diagnosis is essentially clinical and relies on fever for at least 5 consecutive days plus four out of five other criteria:

1. Conjunctivitis — bilateral
2. Oral changes — swollen, red or cracked lips, 'strawberry' tongue and mucosal erythema
3. Peripheral extremity changes — erythema, oedema and desquamation of the hands and feet (desquamation is often a late feature, i.e. after 10 days)
4. Rash — polymorphous
5. Cervical lymphadenopathy — this only occurs in 50–70% and very often can be only one enlarged tender node

It is necessary to exclude other causes of the above symptoms: e.g. *Streptococcus*, *Staphylococcus*, *Leptospirosis*, rickettsiae, measles and Steven-Johnson syndrome by appropriate investigation.

Recommendations have been drawn together in a consensus statement from the 3rd International Kawasaki Disease symposium. For effective treatment diagnosis should be made within 10 days of the onset of fever. The infant / child should receive:

1. Intravenous immunoglobulins — 2 g/kg over 8–12 hours

2. High-dose aspirin — 30–100 mg/kg/day, for 14 days or until the fever remits, then continued as a low dose 3–5 mg/kg/day until cardiological assessment at 6–8 weeks

The child requires initial cardiological investigation with ECG and echocardiography at presentation, looking for evidence of coronary artery dilatation, aneurysm formation, pericarditis and myocarditis. I would follow this with a repeat echocardiogram a fortnight later and at 8 weeks. If normal at 8 weeks, it is highly unlikely that macroscopic dilatation will occur subsequently. Aspirin can be stopped at this point. If abnormalities persist, regular echocardiography should be carried out and low-dose aspirin continued.

Prior to immunoglobulin and aspirin therapy, coronary artery aneurysm formation was in the order of 20–25%, and is more likely in those with high thrombocytosis, leucocytosis, a younger age and prolonged fever. A major study in the UK suggested that immunoglobulin administration within the first 10 days of onset may not actually reduce this figure by a great margin. Other studies suggest dramatic reduction in morbidity and mortality. It may be that immunoglobulins and aspirin reduce the severity (i.e. the diameter of coronary aneurysms) and speed up the resolution of the aneurysms. Mortality in this country is 2–4% and death usually occurs within the first 3 months. Mortality in Japan is only around 0.1%. These huge differences in mortality rates may be in part due to the under treatment of the condition in the UK, but may also be because i.v. immunoglobubin is less effective in UK disease (? due to a different aetiology or because of a different donor population for the production of immunoglobin). For those with persistent coronary artery dilatation, I would seek the long-term follow up of a paediatric cardiologist, and at an appropriate age, an adult cardiologist.

REFERENCES

Akagi T et al 1992 Outcome of coronary artery aneurysms after Kawasaki disease. J Pediatrics 689–693
BPSU annual report 1992
Dhillon R et al 1993 Management of Kawasaki disease in the British Isles. Arch Dis Child 69: 631–638
In: T J David (ed) Recent advances in paediatrics 11: Churchill Livingstone, Edinburgh

Management of cystic fibrosis

Q. Routine neonatal screening has revealed that the first child of a young couple is homozygous for the cystic fibrosis gene. The diagnosis is confirmed at 6 weeks by a sweat test. How would you manage this asymptomatic infant?

I would first take time to explain the diagnosis to both parents. Many people have heard a little about cystic fibrosis but, although relatively common, not many of the general public are aware of the implications of the disease. I would tell them about the important respiratory and gastrointestinal manifestations of the disease, stressing the improving prognosis for children, especially with early treatment. I have been fortunate enough to work with a cystic fibrosis team, including a nurse specialist. This is valuable in educating the parents about the disease, as the main points can be repeated on several occasions. I would also arrange for the family to meet the physiotherapist, dietician and social worker at an early stage.

Physiotherapy should be started early, despite the lack of symptoms. This is thought to improve the prognosis of respiratory disease and also allows the parents to learn the technique and start a routine. Physiotherapy should be twice daily, or more frequently if the child becomes symptomatic. In the infant, physiotherapy will involve gentle manual percussion and vibration. As the child gets older, postural drainage may be helpful and, by mid-childhood, the patient may be able to cooperate with the forced expiratory technique. This allows physiotherapy to be independent of assistance in later childhood. Vigorous exercise, and a healthy cry in the infant, also help to clear secretions.

Pancreatic enzyme supplements should be started soon after diagnosis. Enteric-coated microsphere preparations are currently used. Enzyme release is dependent on pH and occurs when the spheres reach the duodenum. In the infant the spheres can be taken out of the capsule and the amount given is titrated according to the nature of the stool consistency. Peri-anal erythema and skin breakdown may be due to excessive pancreatic enzymes. Exposure of the skin and reduction of the dose usually allow healing.

Diet is another important aspect and the dietician should be involved. *Vitamin supplements* will be required since fat-soluble vitamins are poorly absorbed. Vitamins A, D and E should be given in a water miscible form. Vitamin K is not usually required, but may be necessary in the older child with a prolonged prothrombin time. Weight gain should be carefully monitored, since failure to thrive is a common problem in cystic fibrosis. When weaned, the child will need a diet high in calories with a normal protein content. Glucose polymer supplements may be helpful in the older child.

Antibiotics shoud be given if the infant has symptoms of chest infection. The most common causative organism in the young infant is *Staphylococcus aureus* and is responsive to flucloxacillin. *Haemophilus influenzae* may also affect the young child and amoxycillin will usually clear the organism; however, it is important to realise that 15% of haemophilus organisms are resistant to amoxycillin and the antibiotic should be changed if there is no response to treatment. Oral antibiotics should be given in large doses for a period of a month if chest infection is apparent. Intravenous antibiotics may be required initially if the child is unwell at presentation. *Pseudomonas aeruginosa* uncommonly colonises the young child, but may be a significant problem in the older child.

The role of *prophylactic antibiotics* in the asymptomatic child is less clear. It has been suggested that continuous prophylactic flucloxacillin from diagnosis improves clinical progress in the first 2 years of life, with lower frequency of cough and shorter, less frequent hospital admissions.

The management of this newly diagnosed child with cystic fibrosis would not be complete without counselling the parents about future pregnancies. The inheritance of cystic fibrosis is autosomal recessive. The parents should be told that there is a 1 in 4 chance that a future child will have cystic fibrosis. If the gene mutation has been identified in the child, it is possible to screen antenatally and offer termination in future pregnancies if the fetus is affected. Gene probes are used to detect the gene mutation on chorionic villus biopsy material.

Asthma guidelines

Q1. What are the latest guidelines for the management of asthma in childhood?

The British Thoracic Society (BTS) guidelines (1993) are a revised statement on the diagnosis and management of asthma in adults and children. Input for the document has come from the BTS, the BPA, the RCP of London, the RCGP and others. Its aim is to provide a consensus on the recognition and effective treatment of asthma in the UK to minimise morbidity and mortality from this very common chronic inflammatory condition of the airways.

In essence, the document gives a stepwise management approach to treatment, starting at a level appropriate to the severity of the disease. Success is measured by monitoring: symptoms by day and night, including peak expiratory flow rates (PEFR); the number of days off nursery or school; the participation in everyday activities and sport; and the need for relief medication.

In children particularly, it is essential to select the correct method of administration of anti-asthma medication to maximise drug deposition at the site of efficacy, i.e. the lungs. Great emphasis is placed on the use of large volume spacer devices for all children, certainly below the age of 5, if not using nebulised medication.

Essentially there are five steps to management:

1. Occasional use of relief bronchodilators: Not needing to use more than once a day, on a prn basis.
2. Regular inhaled anti-inflammatory agents: i.e. sodium cromoglycate 10–20 mg t.d.s. plus relief bronchodilators on a prn basis. I would normally give a 6–8 week trial of sodium cromoglycate and assess benefit after this time.
3. Use of inhaled steroids: Beclomethasone or budesonide 50–200 µg b.d. plus intermittent β_2 agonists.
4. Use of high-dose inhaled steroids: Beclomethasone or budesonide 400–800 µg daily plus intermittent β_2 agonists. A trial of regular b.d. long-acting β_2 agonists is worthwhile, especially if nocturnal cough/wheeze or exercise-induced symptoms.
5. High-dose inhaled steroids plus bronchodilators: Beclomethasone or budesonide at 800 µg/day plus the use of slow-release xanthines or nebulised β_2 agonists.

Regular review of treatment is essential and if well controlled, a step down the treatment ladder is attempted. A rescue course of oral steroids may be needed at any step if symptoms are temporarily out of control (prednisolone 1–2 mg/kg, maximum 40 mg/day for 3–5 days).

Gastro-enterology and infection

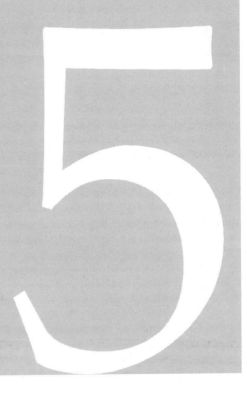

5

Crohn's disease

Q. A 12 year-old boy presents with a history suggestive of Crohn's disease. This is confirmed by biopsy. He has had bilateral knee pain for the past year, for which no cause had been found. How would you treat him?

If he has been previously investigated for his joint pains with no cause found, I would suggest that the arthralgia is secondary to the inflammatory bowel disease and would expect it to improve with treatment of the underlying problem. In the meantime, I would provide symptomatic relief with simple analgesics such as paracetamol.

I would initially check his haemoglobin level and give a blood transfusion if anaemia is confirmed. Further investigation of the bowel will be unnecessary if histological evidence has been found. However, it is important to identify the sites of disease by contrast medium studies if this has not already been done.

Drug treatment is dependant on the site of bowel affected. For all sites of disease I would start by introducing *corticosteroids*. I would begin with a dose of 1 mg/kg/day and continue for 4–6 weeks. If the disease is controlled after that time, I would then gradually reduce the dose over several weeks.

At presentation, I would also start one of the *aminosalicylates*, such as sulphasalazine or mesalazine. Sulphasalazine is a chemical combination of 5-aminosalicylic acid and sulphapyridine and was the first of the group to be used in inflammatory bowel disease. The 5-aminosalicylic acid moiety is the active substance, while the sulphapyridine acts as a carrier to the colon where the molecule is cleaved by bacteria. This explains why sulphasalazine is useful in large but not small bowel disease. The sulphapyridine causes side-effects, including rashes, agranulocytosis and the Stevens-Johnson syndrome.

Mesalazine is 5-aminosalicylic acid with no carrier. It is formulated in a resin which breaks down at the pH of the distal ileum and therefore may be used in small but not large bowel disease. Side-effects are less common because there is no sulphonamide moiety. The tablets are large and younger children may not be able to swallow them.

If the child has evidence of perianal fistulae or abscesses, I would prescribe *metronidazole*. This may also have a beneficial effect in large bowel disease. However, it is known to cause dose-dependant peripheral neuropathy in some patients and should then be stopped.

Nutritional support is important in Crohn's disease. Usually, it is possible to maintain a child on enteral feeds. It may be necessary to give nasogastric feeds at night to maintain the nutritional status while the inflammation is treated. The use of an elemental diet has been advocated and some studies have shown that when used in small bowel disease, clinical remission is comparable with the use of corticosteroids. Symptoms tend to recur when the diet is stopped. An elemental diet is tasteless and most children will only tolerate it if given by nasogastric tube. Occasionally it will be necessary to use total parenteral nutrition in acute disease. Where possible it should be avoided due to the complications of a central venous line, most importantly infection. Poor growth is common in Crohn's disease and is a great concern to the family. Adequate intake of calories is essential.

I would avoid the use of antimotility drugs which might otherwise be used to relieve the diarrhoea. They may cause paralytic ileus and megacolon in severe disease.

Surgery is required in some cases, either if the acute disease causes perforation or if the disease is persistent and recurring. Unfortunately, Crohn's disease tends to recur in the remaining bowel, especially in extensive disease.

If the disease does not improve or is chronically active, it may be necessary to continue corticosteroid treatment for prolonged periods. I would try an alternate day regimen, since this reduces the effect of steroids on linear growth. Immunosuppressants such as azathioprine may be used in cases resistant to therapy. This would have a steroid-sparing effect in extensive disease, but may increase the long-term risk of malignant disease.

Once remission is induced, the drugs should be withdrawn gradually. Unlike ulcerative colitis, there is no role for maintenance drugs, since they have not been proven effective.

Constipation

Q1. Constipation is a common problem in paediatric outpatients. How do you manage these children?

Constipation is defined as the passage of infrequent and sometimes painful stools and is a symptom rather than a disease. Very often the diagnosis only comes to light when a child (or parent) complains of soiling or encopresis due to overflow, although constipation may have been present for months or even years. In the vast majority, no underlying organic cause exists, but must be excluded by appropriate investigation.

Causes include:

1. A normal variation — 'one man's constipation may be another man's diarrhoea'.
2. Lack of dietary fibre/poor fluid intake—these two factors probably are not as important in paediatric constipation as in adults, and modification of diet is difficult to implement, but this should not prevent attempted adjustment, with the advice of the dietician.
3. Failure to develop a regular bowel habit. The causes are multifactorial, but include: over zealous toilet training by parents; painful defaecation; avoidance of the 'call to stool' and a toilet phobia.
4. Anatomical causes — anal fissures are common and lead to stool retention. Hirschsprung's disease is uncommon and produces constipation from birth. These children do not as a rule develop overflow incontinence and rarely have abdominal pain, but have abdominal distension and an empty rectum on PR examination.
5. Hypotonia — hypothyroidism, either congenital or acquired and myopathies.
6. Drugs — e.g. iron preparations, decongestants, antacids (containing calcium or aluminium) and opiates.

Treatment is dependent on age of the child. Infants very often have decreased stool frequency on changing from breast to bottle milk and on weaning. This is normal and requires no treatment other than parental education. However, if constipation is suspected, I would advise simple measures such as adding fruit to the diet or brown sugar to milk feeds. Addition of osmotic and stimulant laxatives may be required short term.

In older children the use of laxatives with modification of the diet is usually effective. My first choice would be lactulose, followed by the addition of senna 10 days later. By holding off senna initially, by the time it is introduced hopefully the stools are softened and therefore less painful when passed.

In children who are grossly constipated, in whom laxatives have been tried with an unsuccessful outcome, a rapid result can be gained by using Picolax, a sodium picosulphate/magnesium citrate combination. In this manner, the problem may be rectified without having to use methods from the 'bottom' end which can further traumatise an already anxious and fearful child. Having said that, occasionally suppositories or enemata may be used in children with hard impacted faeces in the rectum. Avoidance of phosphate enemas in the under 3s is advised to prevent raised serum phosphate levels. The use of manual evacuation is rarely if ever justified in my opinion.

In a child with a megarectum, disimpaction is simply the first step on the road to regular bowel habit. Once the large bowel is emptied of hard faeces, continuation with stimulant and osmotic laxatives is justified to prevent re-accumulation. This may be necessary for many months to allow time for the bowel to contract down to a normal diameter.

The establishment of a regular toilet pattern is an essential component of treatment. This may well be the most difficult part of constipation management in children who associate the toilet with pain and anger from parents. The parents must learn to adopt a less rigid and less demanding approach to the child's toileting. Positive reinforcement engenders enthusiasm and motivation. Sitting the child on the toilet after mealtimes and making it an enjoyable and fun experience will lead to long-term success.

Q2. Have you heard of biofeedback training in the treatment of chronic constipation?

An article in *Archives of Diseases in Childhood* in 1993, written from Amsterdam, suggested biofeedback as a useful therapeutic approach in children with constipation. By means of manometric anal probes and electromyography of the external anal sphincter, defaecation dynamics are recorded during simulated defaecation. The children are taught to recognise the sensation of rectal fullness and to accomplish relaxation of the external anal sphincter.

The group had complete success in 55% (15 out of 29 patients, aged 5–16 years) and incomplete success in the majority of the others. Although I have no experience of these practices, on paper the techniques employed look extremely encouraging. However, it is obviously a very time consuming and labour intensive programme and I wonder about its use in the routine management of constipation in the outpatient department!

REFERENCES

Benninga M A et al 1993 Biofeedback training in chronic constipation. Arch Dis Child 68: 126–129
Clayden G S 1992 Management of chronic constipation. Arch Dis Child 67: 340–344

Chronic diarrhoea

Q1. A GP refers a child with a label of chronic diarrhoea. You see her in outpatients. Tell me how you would proceed.

Chronic diarrhoea is a fairly common reason for a child to be referred to outpatients and is generally defined as the passage of loose stools for more than 2 weeks. I would first establish that the child's symptoms fit this definition before accepting the label.

There are many causes and a thorough history and examination together with certain simple investigations will often yield the diagnosis and save many such children from unnecessary invasive procedures. As I obtain clues from my history and examination, I would review in my mind the features of specific conditions.

The *age* of the child is an important consideration since there are certain conditions which specifically affect younger children. In this regard, I would consider toddler's diarrhoea, secondary disaccharidase deficiency and cow's milk protein intolerance. *Toddler's diarrhoea* is seen in well-children aged 6 months to 2 years, though it can sometimes persist up to the age of 5 years. I would ensure that the parents confirm that the child's general health is good and, as with all causes of diarrhoea, I would make a careful enquiry about the nature of the stool. In toddler's diarrhoea, visibly undigested food will be passed, hence the term 'peas and carrots diarrhoea'. Examination will reveal a normal child and the growth chart will confirm normal weight gain. Once I am satisfied that these features have been established all that I would do is to send stool samples for microbiological examination to exclude a covert infective cause such as giardiasis. The cause of this condition is not fully understood although failure to chew food adequately and rapid gastrointestinal transit time have been implicated.

Secondary disaccharidase deficiency (usually lactase) is another common cause of an episode of chronic diarrhoea in infants and I would look for a history of a precipitating attack of gastroenteritis. Temporary withdrawal of milk and if necessary other carbohydrate-containing foods from the diet should improve the symptoms. *Cow's milk protein intolerance* is a much rarer cause of diarrhoea in infants and can sometimes resemble toddler's diarrhoea, although food particles are absent from the stools. Tests for this condition are complicated and therefore if the diagnosis is suspected, milk is empirically withdrawn from the diet and improvement in symptoms is usually taken to establish the diagnosis clinically. Small amounts of milk accidentally ingested thereafter may induce an acute reaction such as vomiting, diarrhoea, urticaria and bronchospasm. Occasionally, chronic exposure may cause severe failure to thrive, rectal bleeding and hepatosplenomegaly due to an immunological reaction to milk protein.

Three conditions which may present at any age in childhood are giardiasis, coeliac disease and cystic fibrosis. These conditions often have features of malabsorption so I would make a specific enquiry about the passage of offensive, pale, fatty stools which float and may be difficult to flush away. Giardiasis is probably an under-diagnosed cause of chronic diarrhoea and should be especially considered if there has been exposure to institutions such as day nurseries, or over-crowded, deprived accommodation, holiday camps or foreign travel. The condition is caused by the flagellate protozoan, Giardia lamblia, which primarily affects the duodenum and upper jejunum. It produces offensive fatty motion due to secondary disaccharidase deficiency and therefore may mimic coeliac disease. Faeces taken during acute diarrhoea may show the trophozoite of Giardia on microscopy. A patient with chronic giardiasis may have formed or semi-formed stools (and may therefore be asymptomatic) and the diagnostic cysts are more difficult to obtain so three stool samples collected on different days are usually examined. Duodenal aspiration or examination of a jejunal biopsy (which may show villous atrophy as well as parasitic cysts) is necessary in a few children to establish the diagnosis. Metronidazole is the drug of choice.

Both *cystic fibrosis* and *coeliac disease* have an incidence of approximately 1:2000 and may present in similar ways. A child with cystic fibrosis may have a history of recurrent chest infections or chest symptoms and will usually have a normal or even excessive appetite. A child with coeliac disease will usually have symptoms which date from the introduction of gluten-containing foods and will usually appear miserable with a poor appetite and abdominal distension. The child may have a history of mouth ulcers (as with Crohn's disease). Although presentation is usually at 5–7 months, symptoms may commence at any age.

I would consider *inflammatory bowel disease* as a possible cause if there is a history of bloody or mucous diarrhoea or significant abdominal pain, oral signs including ulceration or anal disease or an abdominal mass (Crohn's).

Two drug-related causes are *laxative abuse* (which I would specifically enquire about where appropriate such as in older girls with features to suggest psychological disease) and *pseudomembranous colitis*. Pseudomembranous colitis presents as diarrhoea and abdominal pain and sometimes fever occurring during or even some weeks after a course of broad-spectrum antibiotics, especially amoxycillin and cephalosporins. (The condition was strongly linked to clindamycin but this antibiotic is now rarely used systemically.) Despite the fact that the condition is a colitis, a history of bloody stools is often not obtained. It is especially seen in children with systemic disease such as malignancy or uraemia and is caused by the anaerobic Gram-positive bacillus *Clostridium difficile*, which produces an exotoxin which damages the colon. I would establish the diagnosis by demonstrating the toxin or the organism in the stool and I would treat the condition with either metronidazole or vancomycin orally.

Chronic diarrhoea may be a manifestation of *thyrotoxicosis* and I would enquire about weight loss associated with a good appetite and heat intolerance. I would then look for other signs such as a resting tachycardia, eye signs (especially lid-lag), and a goitre with a palpable thrill or a bruit.

Finally, I would keep at the back of my mind that chronic diarrhoea may also be the presenting symptom of various psychological problems including factitious illness.

During the examination, as well as looking for specific clues, I would look for features of dehydration (such as dry mucous membranes, reduced skin turgor, sunken eyes, hypotension and a sunken anterior fontanelle in babies). If confirmed I would admit the child for intravenous rehydration. Also, features of significant systemic upset such as an abnormal growth chart or emaciation would necessitate admission.

Q2. OK, I'll stop you there. How would you investigate this patient?

This would depend upon the age of the patient, the nature of the stools, the presence of any significant systemic symptoms, the presence of any abnormal signs and the growth chart. It would be reasonable in many cases as an initial assessment to arrange stool examination (and where appropriate multiple samples and a laxative screen), a full blood count and ESR, urea & electrolytes, serum albumin and thyroid function tests. Other investigations to consider would be small bowel aspiration and/or biopsy, sigmoidoscopy with biopsy and a sweat test. In addition, in certain cases, I would use admission of the child to hospital as an investigation to witness stool nature and frequency and also to assess abnormal behaviour and possible laxative abuse.

Tips

- This question is so broad that a structured, logical and reasonably comprehensive response is a tall order. A question of this sort will often be 'the opener' in the viva; the demonstration of solid competence when it comes to dealing with common outpatient problems will score very highly and set the tone for the rest of your time.

- In our experience, the examiner may interrupt you once he or she is satisfied that you are dealing with the problem sensibly and start to 'feed' you specific details. It is important that you state that admission to hospital may be an important step in investigating the problem (though not necessarily at the first visit). The final diagnosis that the examiner has 'in his mind' and wants you to chase will often be an unusual end-point such as laxative abuse or thyrotoxicosis.

Liver transplantation

Q1. What do you know about liver transplantation in children?

Paediatric orthotopic liver transplantation has become accepted practice in Britain over the past 10 years and should now be considered at an early stage in any child with life-threatening hepatic disease. In suitable cases, the potential benefits of this major procedure are far ranging, including improved survival, growth and development.

The longest surviving recipient remains well more than 20 years after transplantation (Whitington et al 1991). The overall success rates are also generally very favourable especially since the introduction of better immunosuppressants, modern tissue typing techniques and improved organ availability.

The donors are generally children (or in some cases adults) who have brain death whilst on a ventilator. This is usually in the context of severe trauma or major intracranial disease without significant damage to other vital organs. The donor is blood and tissue typed and tested for transmissible infections such as viral hepatitis and HIV.

Liver transplantation was originally carried out in children with *chronic liver disease*, generally cirrhosis, and this may be related to:

— *metabolic defects* such as Wilson's disease, 1-α-trypsin deficiency, cystic fibrosis, haemochromatosis, tyrosinaemia or galactosaemia
— *structural genetic defects* such as biliary atresia
— *post-necrotic cirrhosis* such as neonatal hepatitis, chronic aggressive hepatitis, drugs and poisons.

It is also increasingly being used to treat *fulminant liver failure*, such as in Reye syndrome, drug-related (such as paracetamol or halothane) or fulminant viral hepatitis.

Occasionally, liver transplantation is used in certain liver-based metabolic diseases where liver function is not gravely affected but damage to other vital organs is life-threatening. These include familial hypercholesterolaemia, Crigler-Najjar syndrome, urea cycle defects and factor VIII or protein C deficiency. It also has a limited role in the management of some liver tumours.

The timing of liver transplantation is an immensely complex issue governed by a number or factors such as organ availability, geography and financial constraints as well as clinical assessment. In chronic liver disease various clinical indicators in relation to the underlying condition and age of the child may be used, such as INR >1.4, refractory ascites or encephalopathy, GI bleeding, growth retardation or major risk of hepatocellular carcinoma (e.g. in tyrosinaemia).

Acute liver failure is potentially reversible with full recovery (the liver has an immense capacity for regeneration as long as active disease has abated and adequate hepatic mass remains). However, the mortality without transplantation is 90% if the INR is >4.0 and 100% if >6 (Chiyende & Mowat 1992). Four of the 7 children with severe acute liver failure (INR >4) transplanted in 1988–1991 have survived with a median follow-up of 18 months. Any child with acute liver failure with encephalopathy or an INR >1.6 not corrected by i.v. vitamin K should be referred for consideration for transplantation (Chiyende & Mowat 1992).

Q2. Do you know anything about survival after liver transplantation?

The sucess rates following liver transplantation are generally promising, especially in relation to the diseases for which they are undertaken. Analysis of the first 100 children transplanted at the King's/Cambridge unit (between 1983 and 1990) gave an overall survival rate of 65% (Salt et al 1992). More recent figures have shown a 1-year survival of 86% with 5-year survival rates of 64–78%.

Survival in children under 1 year is also high with 1-year rates of 88% in the Birmingham unit (Beath et al 1993). The use of reduction hepatectomy where only part of the liver from an older child or even adult is transplanted has increased organ availability for this age group.

Q3. What do you know about the complications?

Even under the best circumstances, between 10 and 15% of children will die within 3 months of transplantation and there is a significant continuing mortality as well as morbidity. Peri-operatively, the child is at great risk from a combination of major surgery and the effects of the disease that has led to the transplantation. Specific surgical complications include primary non-functioning of the graft, anastomotic leaks or strictures/stenosis from biliary or vascular sites and hepatic vascular thrombosis.

Immunosuppression is required and a commonly used protocol is prednisolone, cyclosporin and azathioprine with prednisolone on a reducing regimen and being discontinued after 3 months and azathioprine being discontinued after 1 year. Cyclosporin is continued indefinitely. Opportunistic infection is therefore a major risk and will affect virtually all patients at some stage. These range from systemic bacterial infection (faecal or pseudomonas), viral infection (EBV and CMV are common late complications), fungal or even protozoal.

Even with close matching of the blood group and tissue antigens of the donor and recipient and immunosuppressive therapy, rejection is a significant problem. This may be acute (which may present with a very similar clinical picture to fulminant infection) or chronic (which is heralded by insidious deterioration of the LFTs).

Up to 40% of recipients need re-transplantation, usually for chronic rejection, hepatic vascular thrombosis or primary non-functioning.

Q4. Why do you think a general paediatrician should know about hepatic transplantation?

Perhaps the most important reason why I keep myself briefed in advancing but rather super-specialised areas such as hepatic transplantation is because the early recognition and referral of suitable cases is often vital to long-term success. This applies to acute cases as well as in chronic liver disease. For example, biliary atresia accounts for over 50% of children transplanted in most centres and there is evidence that diagnosis has been delayed in many cases. It is therefore important to recognise that even mild conjugated hyperbilirubinaemia always implies significant hepatobiliary disease in children.

I would be involved in the general pre-transplantation care of children with chronic disease, including ensuring that they had received a full immunisation programme (including against various viruses, *Streptococcus pneumoniae* and *Haemophilus influenzae*) and supervising their growth and nutrition. Careful counselling of both the child and his or her family is vital and it is important to ensure that expectations are not inappropriately high or low.

Finally, I may at some time be involved in the rather distressing process of caring for the family of a patient who is a potential donor. Again, careful counselling is critical though I feel that successful donation may represent a positive step for the donor's family as well as for the recipient.

Tip

■ You should regard this as a gift of a question as it allows you to steer the discussion into any number of areas that you may be well-up on from hepatology, biochemistry, emergency paediatrics and infection to ethics and social medicine.

REFERENCES

Beath S V et al 1993 Successful liver transplantation in babies under 1 year. Br Med J 307: 825–882
Chiyende J, Mowat A P 1992 Liver transplantation. Arch Dis Child 67: 1124–1127
Salt A et al 1992 Liver transplantation in 100 children: the Cambridge and King's College Hospital series. Br Med J 304: 416–421

Failure to thrive

Q1. What do you understand by the term 'failure to thrive'?

Failure to thrive is a descriptive term which implies that a child has a rate of growth that fails to meet the expected potential for a child of that age. The word 'failure' is, perhaps, unfortunate, since it may signify to the carer that inadequate parenting is responsible for the poor growth of the child. Failure to thrive has many causes and may be a combination of nutritional problems, poor general health and psychosocial deprivation. It is important to identify these children, since it may have a persistent effect on final height and intellectual development.

Q2. So, how would you identify these children and which ones would you investigate?

GPs and health visitors have an important role in screening for growth. Plotting weight and head circumference on growth charts is routine for most infants. Although the centile for birthweight is usually used to indicate the growth potential, it has been suggested that a weight at 6 weeks would be a more accurate predictor of final growth centiles, when maternal nutrition has less of an effect on weight.

A child may be referred to the hospital when his/her weight is below the 3rd, or sometimes 10th, centile according to the growth charts designed by Tanner and Whitehouse. It is important to check previous weights, since a child may be constitutionally small, but thriving. A single measurement may be of little value, whereas 'falling through the centiles' is significant. Ideally the child should be measured on the same scales on subsequent visits, naked in a younger child and with minimal clothing in an older child. Note should be made of the child's state of dress.

The Tanner growth charts were designed from the measurements of relatively small numbers of children and therefore may not give a true picture of the 'average' weight and height at present. New growth charts have been designed to take account of a much larger population in a more modern setting. However, actual height or weight may still not be a good indication of failure to thrive, particularly in an older child when height velocity is a more relevant measurement.

There are many children who will be small. By definition 10% of children are below the 10th centile. It is important to identify those children who are constitutionally small to avoid unnecessary investigation. Normal short children may have had a low birthweight due to prematurity, when 'catch up' growth is reduced or may have lower growth potential due to small parents. I always plot the heights of both parents on the child's growth chart so that mid-parental height, and consequently the child's growth potential, can be seen. In a normal small child I would reassure the parents but follow the child for a few months to check that growth remains along the centiles.

The most common cause of failure to thrive, especially in infancy, is *poor feeding*. Again, this should be identified early to avoid investigation. I would want a detailed history of food intake, including amount of milk offered and taken in an infant and the type of food eaten, including snacks, in an older child. While talking to the mother, an impression of her emotional state, self-perception as a parent and attitude towards feeding should be gained. It may be found that the whole family has an unhealthy diet; that the mother herself has an eating disorder, such as anorexia nervosa; or that the mother believes that her child is allergic to certain foods and therefore eliminates them from the diet.

If there is no indication that the child is constitutionally small or has inadequate nutrition to grow, failure to thrive may be either organic or inorganic. About 30–40% of children with true failure to thrive have an *organic* cause. This may be due to chronic illness, e.g. congenital heart disease or chronic renal failure, and these should be found on clinical history and examination. Any other child may warrant further investigations and these should be used selectively depending on the history. It should not be assumed that a child from a deprived background is failing to thrive due to neglect. Sometimes a period of time admitted to hospital may be required to assess the feeding pattern of a child. This should be carefully considered since hospital admission may disempower the mother and cause considerable guilt.

A child may be found to grow well in hospital and the social circumstances then need to be included in the differential diagnosis.

In summary, I would only investigate those children with a reduced growth velocity after careful measurement and I would direct the investigations according to the history obtained.

Dehydration and rehydration

Q. How would you assess and treat dehydration in a child?

Assessment of dehydration is a clinical skill that is carried out many times a day in general practice and in the casualty department of hospitals. The most important decisions are:

— does this child need hospital admission for rehydration?
— does this child need intravenous fluid replacement?

Should the answer to these questions be yes, then the problem arises of how much and what sort? Dehydration can be classified in two ways:

1. Tonicity: hypotonic
                       isotonic
                       hypertonic dehydration
2. Natraemic state: hyponatraemic serum Na^+ <130 mmol/1
                       isonatraemic serum Na^+ 130–150 mmol/1
                       hypernatraemic serum Na^+ > 150 mmol/1

The categories are not interchangeable.

Severity of dehydration is usually based on percentage body weight loss as mild (<5%), moderate (5–9%) and severe (>10%). The most accurate way to determine this is by knowing a recent body weight prior to the onset of the current illness and comparing with admission weight. However, aspects of the history and examination must be elicited to confirm or determine your judgement. From the history, the frequency of micturition is very relevant. In mild dehydration, urine output is essentially normal, in moderate dehydration it is reduced and concentrated and with severe dehydration, urine output is minimal and the last urine output may have been many hours previously. Of course, with the clinical picture of dehydration with inappropriate or excess urine output, diabetes mellitus, diabetes insipidus and chronic renal failure must be thought of and excluded by appropriate investigation.

Clinical signs of dehydration include:

Mild (<5%)	Alert, but restless child with normal BP, heart rate. Moist mucus membranes and normal skin elasticity
Moderate (5–10%)	Dry mucus membranes, sunken eyes and fontanelle (if appropriate) with increased skin turgor
Severe (>10%)	Drowsy, irritable child with cool peripheries, rapid and feeble pulses. Very sunken eyes and markedly increased skin turgor. Coma and unrecordable BP in more severe cases

NB With hypernatraemic dehydration the skin takes on a doughy texture. My *initial investigation and management* would involve:

1. Weigh the child
2. I.V. access: FBC + haematocrit, U & Es + osmolality
3. I.V. PPF/0.9% normal saline 20 ml/kg over 30 minutes if shocked
4. Strict input and output measurement
5. Urine osmolality and electrolytes if severe

Subsequent rehydration should take place over the next 24–48 hours and is dictated by severity and type of dehydration.

a) *Hypotonic dehydration.* I would use either 0.45% or 0.9% N/Saline (80 mmol/l and 156 mmol/l respectively) and give 50% of deficit in the first 8 hours and the remainder over the next 16 hours on top of maintenance fluids and combined losses.
   — Maintenance fluids
      (i) Water   4 ml/kg/hour for the first 10 kg body weight
                          2 ml/kg/hour for the next 10 kg
                          1 ml/kg/hour for the remainder
      (ii) Electrolytes Na^+ 2–3 mmol/kg/24 hours
                          K^+ 2–3 mmol/kg/24 hours
   — Deficit fluids
      e.g. 10% dehydration in a 20 kg child with a sodium of 115 mmol/l
      (i) Water   10% of 20 kg = 2 kg = 2000 ml deficit
                          1000 ml in the first 8 hours
                          1000 ml in the second 16 hours
      (ii) Electrolytes Na^+ in 20 kg child = 115
           Deficit $= [(135-115) \times weight \times 0.6 \text{ (i.e. ECF}^*)] +$
                          (fluid deficit $\times$ 115)
                          $= 20 \times 20 \times 0.6 + 2 \times 115$
                          $= 470$ mmol Na^+

*as majority of Na^+ is in ECF

The child with severe hypotonic dehydration will have a metabolic acidosis, but I would rarely if ever correct this with an infusion of sodium bicarbonate. Electrolyte and fluid correction will bring up the serum pH in a much more physiological manner.

      (iii) Replacement fluids: i.e. urine, stool, vomitus, blood. Fluid should be replaced with like, usually 0.45% or 0.9% N/saline + KCl, in equal volume to the previous 1–4 hours losses, dependent on severity of dehydration

b) *Isotonic dehydration.* Again correction over 24 hours is acceptable and I would use 0.45% saline/5% dextrose after initial resuscitation fluids.

c) *Hypertonic dehydration.* I would correct this more slowly, taking 48 hours at least to avoid cerebral oedema and possible seizures. Assessment of dehydration is difficult because the usual clinical signs of severe dehydration may be lacking, i.e. increase in skin turgor, sunken fontanelle. After initial resuscitation I would use either 0.45% N/Saline or 0.18% N/Saline (-32 mmol/l N^+).

Deficit = normal body water – present body water
= (weight $\times$ 0.6 $\times$ osmolality) – weight $\times$ 0.6

In all three types of dehydration, the addition of KCl to the rehydration fluids is titrated against serum K^+ measurement and urine output.

Vomiting in a 3 month old

Q. A 3 month old is referred to you with recurrent vomiting. What are you going to do?

This is an extremely common referral problem of infancy and fortunately, in the vast majority of children, of a non-serious nature. In over 90% the diagnosis will be straightforward *gastro-oesophageal reflux* (GOR), but it is essential to exclude pathological causes by means of thorough history taking, examination and investigation as indicated. Salient features to come out of the history include:

1. Timing of the vomiting — i.e. related or unrelated to feeds. More relevant if not related to feeds.
2. Nature of the vomiting — i.e. poseting or vomiting, effortless, projectile.
3. Nature of the vomitus — i.e. bile-stained, blood-stained, curdled milk. *Bile-stained vomiting is always pathological.*
4. Onset of the vomiting — after 6 weeks of age it is unlikely to be GOR.
5. Is the infant thriving? Simple GOR does not cause failure to thrive.
6. Associated features, e.g. diarrhoea, steatorrhoea, bloody stools, cough.

These questions would then direct me towards the most likely aetiological cause, i.e. GOR, gastrointestinal (congenital hypertrophic pyloric stenosis, cow's milk enteropathy, malrotation with intermittent volvulus, etc.), respiratory (cystic fibrosis, whooping cough), infection, metabolic, etc.

Only if a pathological cause is suspected or the infant is not thriving, would I undertake investigation (except urinalysis to exclude a urinary tract infection). Advice would then be given to minimise GOR. Simple measures would be elevation of the head of the cot, not nursing the baby in a sitting position after feeds as this is the worst anti-reflux position and thickening the feeds with carobel (1 scoop to 100 ml of milk and enlarge the aperture of the teat by means of a longitudinal slit). Together with these measures, Gaviscon can be used on a trial basis.

More contentious measures include the use of H_2-antagonists and nursing the infant in a prone position after feeds and when sleeping. This latter approach is a very effective method of reducing reflux but creates anxiety regarding the increased incidence of sudden infant death syndrome (SIDS).

For GOR a realistic prognostic picture would be that the vomiting settles down by 18 months of age as the child adopts a more upright posture, although a significant proportion will settle down much earlier. I would review the infant in the outpatient department 1 month after starting treatment to assess progress.

In any infant with recurrent vomiting in whom another cause besides simple GOR is possible, or in those with suspected GOR but failing to thrive, I would investigate accordingly at the first consult.

Chronic abdominal pain

Q. What is your strategy for dealing with recurrent abdominal pain in children?

Recurrent abdominal pain (RAP) in childhood is something that I have encountered many times in clinic. Ideally the first consultation requires a 30 minute appointment during which a picture can be gained regarding the nature of the pain, the degree of disruption the pain causes and the ways that the pain is dealt with by patient, family and school. The incidence of RAP in childhood is at least 10% of over 5 year olds and in <10% of these an organic cause is found. Broadly, these organic causes include:

1. Gastrointestinal: gastro-oesophageal   reflux,   gastritis/duodenitis, constipation, inflammatory bowel disease, coeliac disease, gallstones
2. Urological: recurrent UTIs, reflux nephropathy, renal stones
3. Haematological: abdominal crises in sickle cell disease, hypersplenism
4. Miscellaneous: porphyria, Henoch-Schönlein purpura, lead poisoning

Key questions to be asked initially would be:

1. *Location of the pain?* Peri-umbilical pain suggests non-organic causation, whereas epigastric, suprapubic and lateral pain is more likely to be of organic origin.
2. *Timing of the pain?* Post-prandial suggests dyspepsia or constipation. Nocturnal pain suggests duodenitis/duodenal ulceration. Pain starting on Monday mornings (school phobia), pain starting on the death of a pet, moving home or school, divorce or death of a parent, step father moving in (? child sexual abuse) all suggest a non-organic cause.
3. *Any change in bowel frequency?*
4. *Other gastrointestinal disease?* e.g. mouth ulceration, anal fissuring, melaena, nausea and vomiting.
5. *Exacerbating factors?* e.g. cow's milk, fatty foods.
6. *Urinary symptoms?*
7. *Family history?* of RAP, migraine, anxiety disorders
8. *Social circumstances?*

Examination will very often be unrewarding but must be thorough.

Investigation of a child with RAP, as with examination, will most likely be of no diagnostic value. The performance of unpleasant and invasive procedures to exclude organic causes can lead to a spiral situation of more and more ruthless practice in which a child may have MCUGs, upper and lower gastrointestinal endoscopies, laparoscopy, appendicectomy, etc. for non-specific abdominal pain (NSAP).

Investigative procedures must be highly selective and for a child with the suggestion of RAP, I would undertake only urine microscopy and culture at the first clinic appointment. Obviously features of the history and examination may indicate an organic cause and the need for investigation of the appropriate system.

The typical picture of a child with RAP with no organic cause would be a girl with periumbilical pain, lasting from minutes to several hours, occurring intermittently over days and months with nausea and vomiting, pallor and headaches. Anorexia may or may not be a feature. Both the child and parents may believe that there is a cause for the pain, e.g. cancer because an uncle died of a liver tumour recently, or duodenal ulcer because the father has one and it took months for the diagnosis to be made. Underlying anxieties may take many consultations before they come to light. Both child and parents must be taken seriously and criticism must not be levelled at parenting skills. Reasurrance that there is nothing seriously wrong with the child can represent the world being lifted off the family's shoulders. That the child does not need detailed investigation and disruption of a normal lifestyle can have dramatic results. The child can and should go out and ride his/her bike, climb trees, do PE at school like any other child of the same age. Like an adult, a child can feel stress and anxiety and this can manifest itself as real symptoms of pain and vomiting. As adults with anxiety we may combat the problem by wanting to be alone and likewise a child may not want to talk about it, eat or socialise. Involvement of the school, to prevent the child being sent home repeatedly must be undertaken. If there are problems in the home, social services involvement may be advantageous; clinical psychologists may also have a role to play. Reassurance that the abdominal pain should eventually settle down as the child grows up may not always be true, but in the vast majority it will be. Simple analgesia if giving symptomatic relief, can be worthwhile provided it is not in excess. Long-term follow up in clinic may be necessary.

REFERENCES

Apley J 1975 The child with abdominal pains. Blackwells Scientific, Oxford
Marcovitch M 1993 Management of recurrent abdominal pain. Arch Dis Child 69: 409–411

Helicobacter pylori

Q. What do you know about the role of *H. pylori* in paediatric gastroenterology?

Helicobacter pylori is a spiral shaped, Gram-negative, urease-producing bacterium which was previously known as *Campylobacter pylori*. *H. pylori* colonises the mucous layer of the gastric antrum and attaches to surface epithelial cells by pedicles. It does not appear actually to invade these cells. Extensive work has now been carried out investigating its association with duodenal ulcer disease, gastritis, recurrent abdominal pain and non-ulcer dyspepsia, gastric carcinoma and asymptomatic carriage. Although much of the original work related to adult practice, the importance of *H. pylori* in paediatric gastroenterology has now been established.

H. pylori can be detected by a variety of techniques including histologically in gastric biopsy specimens or by adding urea to biopsy specimens and detecting urease activity. *H. pylori* can also be screened for non-invasively by the use of specific serum antibodies or by the urea breath test with ^{13}C or ^{14}C.

The epidemiology of *H. pylori* is interesting. There is a higher prevalence of the organism in lower socioeconomic groups and in underdeveloped countries and colonisation also increases with age. Familial clustering occurs, which suggests person-to-person spread.

Acute infection in adults may be associated with nausea, vomiting, flatulence and anorexia. However, acute infection as with chronic carriage, may also be asymptomatic.

The strongest correlation of *H. pylori* is with *duodenal ulceration* and *chronic gastritis*. Although peptic ulcer disease is much less common in children than in adults, it has become an increasingly recognised entity in recent years. A paediatrician with an interest in gastroenterology would expect to see around two new cases of duodenal ulceration per month. An American study found the prevalence of duodenal ulceration to be 13.7/100 000 in boys by the age of 15 years and showed the incidence in boys to be approximately 4 times greater than that in girls. Duodenal ulceration predominates over gastric ulceration after approximately 6 years of age (in the first 2 years of life they occur with similar frequency). Over 90% of duodenal ulceration in children is associated with the presence of *H. pylori* in the gastric antrum and in general terms, these so-called 'primary' duodenal ulcers do not recur once the *H. pylori* has been eradicated, unless reinfection occurs. Indeed, the finding of duodenal ulceration in a child in the absence of *H. pylori* or non-steroidal analgesic exposure should spur the clinician to exclude other causes such as a pancreatic gastrinoma in the Zollinger-Ellison syndrome.

H. pylori colonisation of the stomach is always associated with *antral gastritis* in children although these children are often asymptomatic. The most controversial area is the proposed relationship between *H. pylori* and chronic or recurrent abdominal pain in childhood. Several studies have investigated this using various methods including prospectively assessing symptoms in children undergoing upper endoscopy and analysing the prevalence of *H. pylori*-specific antibodies in children with recurrent abdominal pain compared with asymptomatic children. The conclusion from these is that there is no evidence that *H. pylori* gastritis is a cause of chronic abdominal pain in childhood.

There are a variety of regimens which can be used to eradicate *H. pylori*, including amoxycillin for 4 weeks together with omeprazole for 2 weeks or amoxycillin and metronidazole for 6 weeks together with bismuth chelate for 1 month.

Future work into *H. pylori* promises to be exciting. There is increasing evidence that *H. pylori* chronic gastritis and its related atrophic effects are associated with increased risk of gastric carcinoma in adults. Work needs to be done to quantify this association and establish the importance of infection in childhood with later development of carcinoma. The role of person-to-person spread is also interesting. A recent article (Webb et al 1994) has again demonstrated the importance of low socioeconomic status and shown that crowding and close contact in childhood is an important determinant of seroprevalence of *H. pylori* in adulthood. This suggests that infection is transmitted directly from one person to another and may be commonly acquired in early life. The possible benefits of treating whole families and other contacts therefore needs to be analysed.

Tip

■ This would be a good 'hot topic' or recent advances question. It always pays to set the scene with some broad background statements and then give an overview of our current understanding of the subject, highlighting what we already know and what is speculation. Try to show that you have a feel for why the topic is relevant to a modern paediatrician and that you are aware of how future developments may modify practice.

REFERENCES

Gormally S, Drumm B 1994 *Helicobacter pylori* and gastrointestinal symptoms. Arch Dis Child 70: 165–166

Webb P M et al 1994 Relation between infection with *Helicobacter pylori* and living conditions in childhood: evidence for person to person transmission in early life. Br Med J 308: 750–753

Pyrexia of unknown origin

Q1. What is your approach to a child with a pyrexia of unknown origin?

Strictly speaking, the definition of 'pyrexia of unknown origin' (PUO) is reserved for those patients who have unexplained pyrexia despite 3 weeks of hospital investigation. However, the term is now often applied to febrile children who remain undiagnosed after 1 week of hospital investigation, and the approach is the same.

Although there is a long list of causes of PUO, I think it helps to remember that in children most cases are due to infection or autoimmune disorders. The *infectious* causes can be further divided into

1. Bacterial (TB, SBE, abscesses, osteomyelitis)
2. Viral (EBV CMV and HIV)
3. Protozoal (malaria, toxoplasmosis)
4. Fungal (histoplasmosis)

Juvenile chronic arthritis (JCA), SLE and inflammatory bowel disease make up most of the *autoimmune* causes. There are also neoplastic causes, such as leukaemia, lymphoma and Wilms' tumour, and miscellaneous causes — Kawasaki's disease, drug fevers and factitious fevers.

With a list like this in mind, I would retake the history concentrating in particular on aspects such as foreign travel (malaria, brucellosis), the health of other family members (tuberculosis, HIV), any pets and their health (psitticosis). Weight loss is important, as is the presence of sweats and rigors (collection of pus, e.g. pelvic abscess of pyelonephritis). Mild diarrhoea may point to gastrointestinal causes, such as inflammatory bowel disease. Arthritis may be part of JCA, but arthralgia may also occur in other autoimmune conditions, or leukaemias. Sporting activities might point to possible diagnoses, e.g. pot-holers are at risk of histoplasmosis, and water sports can give exposure to leptospirosis. Parents do not usually volunteer such information, not knowing of its importance, so it is only by careful retaking of the history that such clues can be detected.

In a similar way, it is vital to re-examine the patient for subtle signs that may initially have been overlooked. Rashes may indicate JCA or SLE. A tick bite may be the portal of entry of typhus, and a rose spot may indicate typhoid fever. Apthous ulcers in the mouth may be a sign of Crohn's disease. If there is any suggestive history, the eyes should be examined for iritis. I would re-examine the child daily for signs such as lymphadenopathy, or stigmata of endocarditis, which may not initially be present.

Q2. How would you investigate such a child?

Again, there is a long list of possible investigations of such a child. But the important thing is to do these in a sensible order, guided by findings from the history and examination.

Initial investigations include FBC, ESR, U&E, LFT, examination of blood film, and blood cultures, plus a chest X-ray. Baseline serology is important including viral titres and titres for atypical organisms such as rickettsia, coxiella, legionella, mycoplasma, and toxoplasma. It is worth asking for baseline serum to be stored for other investigations which may be thought relevent later. Antistreptolysin O titre should be taken, as should autoantibody titres. If tuberculosis is suspected, I would perform a tuberculin test. Swabs of nose and throat should be taken, and urine and stool examined and cultured. Blood cultures should be repeated several times, particularly when temperature is up. Any enlarged lymph node should be considered for biopsy.

If investigations have so far failed to reveal a diagnosis, I would proceed to further *imaging* investigations. Depending on pointers from the history and examination, these might include abdominal ultrasound or CT for collections, intravenous pylorogram and barium studies. More invasive investigations may also be appropriate including lumbar puncture, rectal biopsy, endoscopy with biopsy, bone marrow, liver biopsy, or rarely diagnostic laparotomy.

Occasionally, if a child is deteriorating, it may be necessary to start empirical treatment with antibiotics before the cause of the pyrexia is known. In these cases, it is important to record serial CRP and ESR to help monitor whether treatment is working.

It is usual practice to admit a child for investigation of fever of unknown origin. But once the process of investigation has begun, if the child is not too unwell, it may be appropriate to allow the child home with a temperature chart, whilst results are awaited.

Tip

- ■ A rather general question like this is not too difficult if you have a clearly structured approach. If the examiner has a particular diagnosis in mind, he/she will guide you towards it as your answer progresses.

HIV and AIDS

Q1. How do children become infected with HIV?

In the majority of children, HIV infection is due to *vertical* transmission, i.e. from the mother. The exceptions, haemophiliacs and recipients of blood transfusion, have become much rarer since screening of donated blood.

Around 20–30% of HIV-infected pregnant mothers transmit the infection to their babies. What determines which infants become infected is not known. There is some suggestion that mothers with more severe disease are more likely to transmit the infection, and a recent study found HIV 1 was more likely to be transmitted than HIV 2. The relative contributions of transplacental infection, and infection from the birth canal during delivery are debated; recent data suggest that caesarian section reduces the risk of transmission. There is also evidence that transmission of the virus can occur via breast milk. HIV is found in lymphocytes in the milk. Thus in the UK, HIV-infected mothers are advised not to breastfeed their children. In Africa, however, because of the greater risk of poor nutrition, breastfeeding is advised.

Q2. How is HIV infection diagnosed?

Diagnosing HIV infection in the infant of an infected mother is difficult. Most children born to HIV-infected mothers have maternal anti-HIV IgG antibodies which have been transmitted across the placenta. This is irrespective of whether they are themselves infected. Loss of antibody by 15 months of age indicates that the child is not infected. Persistance of the antibody after 15 months, or rising levels, indicates the child is infected. Earlier diagnosis of HIV infection is possible if a child has IgA anti-HIV antibodies. These do not cross the placenta and so must have been produced by the child in response to infection. Alternatively, if a child has evidence of infection, such as *Pnemocystis carinii* pneumonia, AIDS can be diagnosed before 15 months.

More recently, it has become possible to detect the viral antigen p24 by ELISA (enzyme linked immunosorbant assay). This can be used much earlier (after about 6 weeks) to provide evidence of infection. PCR (polymerase chain reaction), will allow earlier detection of other viral antigens. Culture of the virus from peripheral blood lymphocytes provides another means of diagnosis.

A number of other laboratory markers of HIV infection are now used to provide additional evidence, though they are not diagnostic on their own. T helper lymphocytes with the CD4 cell surface marker (CD4 cells) are reduced in HIV infection. In normal infants the CD4 count is initially very high, dropping to adult values by about 6 years of age. There may also be hypergammaglobulinaemia, or more rarely hypogammaglobulinaemia.

Q3. What about AIDS itself; how does the disease in children differ from that in adults?

About 20% of infants infected with HIV develop symptoms of AIDS in the first year of life. *Pneumocystis carinii* pneumonia (PCP) occurs at a much earlier stage in children than adults. Most infants present with this and deteriorate very rapidly. The majority of infected children, however, do not develop symptoms until age 2 or 3. In these children, the disease progresses in a similar way to that in adults with certain important exceptions.

Lymphoproliferative manifestations such as hepatosplenomegaly and parotid gland enlargement are more common in children. Lymphoid interstitial pneumuonitis (LIP) is an infiltration of the lungs by lymphocytes, almost never seen in adults. Children with LIP present with a gradual onset of tachypnoea, cough and wheeze. They may also be clubbed. Chest X-ray shows a reticulonodular pattern, and if the diagnosis is uncertain, lung biopsy can be performed. Central nervous system involvement in childhood AIDS is characterised by developmental delay or regression and encephalopathy. But unlike adult AIDS where superadded infections or CNS tumours occur, the deterioration in children is thought to be due to the virus itself. In general, neoplasms are much rarer in childhood than adult AIDS.

Q4. What about management of HIV and AIDS?

I think of management in terms of *medical* and *psychosocial*. The essence of medical treatment is to introduce zidovudine at an appropriate time, provide prophylaxis against infection and treat infections rigorously when they occur. Zidovudine is an HIV reverse transcriptase inhibitor which prevents viral RNA being converted into DNA. It has been shown to prolong survival in adults with established AIDS and is recommended for use in children. It was hoped that its earlier use in HIV-positive patients before they developed AIDS might delay disease progression. However, the double-blind Concorde trial shows that this is not so for adults. Early reports from a study in which zidovudine was given prophylactically to pregnant HIV-positive women and their newborn infants indicate this might reduce vertical transmission. Zidovudine has important side-effects, such as marrow supression. Newer antiretroviral agents, such as dideoxycytidine and DDI, are now licensed as alternative agents.

Prophylaxis against PCP with cotrimoxazole is recommended once the CD4 count has fallen below a certain level. A recent study found that many children were developing PCP before they had reached treatment thresholds, so new guidelines are being drawn up. A CD4 count of 2000/μl has been proposed. Bacterial infections are also a common feature of AIDS in children. These include recurrent otitis media and bacterial meningitis.

Immunisation is an important part of medical management. HIV-infected children should receive all the usual immunisations (except killed polio vaccine is used instead of oral live vaccine). The other live vaccines should be given, except for BCG. HIV-positive children should also receive pneumococcal and influenza vaccines.

Providing support for the child with HIV or AIDS and the whole family is very important. Often other family members will be infected with HIV too. A multidisciplinary approach is required, and the co-operation of social workers, health visitors and school teachers is essential.

Endocrinology, growth and renal medicine

6

Does good diabetic control matter?

Q. Does good diabetic control matter in the child?

Children are at high risk of the complications of diabetes mellitus since they have the disease for more years than in adult onset. Severe retinopathy, nephropathy and neuropathy are rarely seen in the paediatric diabetic clinic, but warning signs, such as early retinopathy, hypertension and microalbuminuria may be noted. These may go on to develop into more serious disease if diabetes is poorly controlled.

Control of diabetes in children is difficult. In the younger child, insulin requirements are not usually high (<1 U/kg/day) and vary considerably in the first few months of the disease. The child is understandably reluctant to have injections although these are better tolerated than the stabs required for home monitoring. Monitoring of blood sugars is therefore quite sporadic in many families. In the adolescent, diabetic control is notoriously difficult, partly due to the disease itself (with increased insulin requirements during this rapid phase of growth) and partly due to poor compliance.

Previous trials have not demonstrated a consistent effect of intensive therapy on long-term complications. It has been shown that tight control of diabetes when *microalbuminuria* develops can reverse progression of renal disease. This is important due to the mortality from renal failure in diabetic patients.

Recently, the 'diabetes control and complications trial' research group investigated the effect of intensive treatment on the development of microvascular complications. They studied a large number of patients with insulin-dependant diabetes mellitus between the ages of 13 and 39 for a mean of 6.5 years. However, the trial contained few highly motivated adolescent recruits. These were divided into two groups. The first were put on an intensive therapy regimen, which meant either using an insulin infusion pump or 3 or more daily insulin injections. The dose of insulin was adjusted according to the blood glucose which was monitored at least 4 times a day. The second group were left on conventional therapy, which meant 1 or 2 daily insulin injections, daily self monitoring of blood glucose and education, but usually no daily alteration of insulin dose.

The trial showed a reduction in significant retinopathy of 50%, of microalbuminuria of 35% and of neuropathy of 70%. There was no significant reduction in macrovascular disease, but this was a young population. Only 5% of the intensive therapy group consistently achieved a glycosylated haemoglobin within the normal non-diabetic range. The hazards of intensive therapy were accelerated weight gain and a 3-fold increase in severe hypoglycaemia. The trial found no difference in perceived quality of life between the two groups.

In summary, the trial showed that intensive therapy with feedback and frequent changes in insulin dose reduces the mean glucose level over several years and delays, or possibly prevents, the development of microvascular disease, while increasing the risk of hypoglycaemia. The introduction of this regimen would be unpopular with children due to the frequent injections and blood tests required. The fear of hypoglycaemia is very real in children, who may be unable to recognise the warning signs of low blood sugar in time to correct it. Hypoglycaemia is also an important concern since repeated severe hypoglycaemia will affect IQ as well as impairing central nervous system awareness for future attacks. The direct feedback of glycosylated haemoglobin results to the patients in the intensive group is likely to have had a major effect on blood glucose control. Those in the conventional group missed out on this positive feedback.

While it does seem likely that rigorous diabetic control is important in reducing the complications of diabetes mellitus, it is difficult to ensure compliance in the adolescent age group. Weight gain and risk of hypoglycaemia will have a major effect on lifestyle and confidence in the fragile adolescent diabetic. A multiple injection regimen, e.g. using the pen injectors with changes according to blood glucose monitoring, seems the most reliable way of ensuring good control in the brittle diabetic. It would seem that optimal control with current insulin regimens and frequent feedback of glycosylated haemoglobin results, with education about the necessary changes in insulin dose, might be the ideal method for reducing the long-term complications.

Tip

- The examiner may divert the conversation at key points; e.g. if an important concept such as hypoglycaemia is mentioned or they identify a weakness in the candidate.

REFERENCE

The Diabetes Control and Complications Trial Research Group 1993 The effect of intensive treatment of diabetes on the development and progression of long-term complications in insulin-dependent diabetes mellitus. New Engl J Med 329: 977–986

Diabetic microalbuminuria

Q. What do you know about diabetic microalbuminuria?

A small amount of albumin is lost in the urine of healthy people which can be detected with specialised laboratory techniques (such as radioimmunoassay). The normal albumin excretion rate (AER) is up to about 20 mg in a 24-hour collection. Microalbuminuria is defined by consensus as an AER above normal but below that detectable by Albustix (30–300 mg per 24 hour collection or 20–200 µg/min in adults). Workers are attempting to produce figures in relation to age or surface area, which may be more appropriate for younger children.

There is now convincing evidence that microalbuminuria in patients with diabetes is predictive of the later development of nephropathy. Various studies have suggested that over 80% of those with persistent microalbuminuria will go on to develop overt renal disease and the rate of increase in albumin excretion is estimated at between 20 and 40% per year. The interval for the progression from the onset of microalbuminuria to overt proteinuria is therefore around 13–18 years. Microalbuminuria can now be screened for using specialised urine strips ('Micral-Test') before laboratory analysis is undertaken.

Longitudinal studies have shown that 40–50% of patients with insulin-dependent diabetes develop nephropathy which therefore means that around half of them are protected from progressive renal damage (the reasons for this are not fully understood). In addition, the results from DCCT have confirmed the clinical view that long-term 'tight' diabetic control does reduce the rate of progression to clinically significant renal impairment.

Evidence suggests that microalbuminuria presents at a reversible stage of nephropathy and may prove to be a valuable method of identifying patients, including children, who are at particular risk of renal disease. The possible management options for these children once they have been identified are:

1. Extra vigilance in glycaemic control
2. Careful screening for and treatment of hypertension
3. Protein-restricted diet (probably not appropriate)
4. ACE inhibitors; have renal-protective effects, even in the absence of hypertension, and multicentre trials to investigate the potential benefits of these drugs in diabetic children are being planned.

In summary, although clinical diabetic renal disease is extremely rare in children, its earliest detectable manifestation, namely microalbuminuria, may be found if it is specifically screened for. This is an area which clearly requires further evaluation but it is hoped that it will prove to be an effective method of directing intensified management in particular cases in order successfully to reduce the number who progress to end-stage renal failure.

A newly diagnosed diabetic

Q. How would you manage a newly diagnosed diabetic who presents with polyuria?

The majority of diabetic children have only minor symptoms at diagnosis, rather than ketoacidosis, and prolonged hospital admission should not be required. The important aims of the admission are to initiate treatment and education.

Treatment is intended to provide adequate nutrition and insulin in order to prevent the symptoms of polydipsia and polyuria, while avoiding hypoglycaemia and allowing normal growth and development. Education about diabetes should be part of the immediate management.

If the child is reasonably well on admission, with no ketonuria, I would start an insulin regimen where the total daily dose is approximately 0.5–1 U/kg. The actual dose would depend on the level of hyperglycaemia and I would use the higher dose if a small amount of ketones is present in the urine. I would start with two-thirds of the dose as medium-acting insulin and one-third as short-acting insulin. I would prescribe two-thirds of the total daily dose before breakfast and the remaining third before the evening meal.

Both the child and the parents need to be shown how to give the insulin subcutaneously. Some children will adapt to giving their own injections rapidly, while others will be unable to manage the difficult process of mixing the insulin, accurately measuring the dose and actually injecting it. I feel both parents should be taught and allowed to practise the method before discharge, in case one parent is not at home. At a later stage, when the dose is stable, it will be possible to use a pen injection device, which uses a defined mixture of short- and medium-acting insulins. This has proved to be more accurate and easier for most children to use. The child should be taught to rotate the injection sites, in order to prevent lipohypertrophy.

The insulin dose is likely to need some adjustment in the early stages of the disease. Regular blood sugars should be checked before meals, using reagent sticks and the insulin dose changed according to these results. For example, if the sugars are consistently high in the late morning, I would increase the short-acting insulin in the morning dose, whereas if the blood sugar is low in the late afternoon, I would reduce the morning medium-acting insulin.

The insulin requirements may be quite low once the initial raised blood glucose is corrected, due to residual functioning pancreatic tissue. Indeed, there may be a period where the child requires no insulin at all, the so-called 'honeymoon' phase. For this reason, it is necessary to monitor the blood glucose frequently initially. However, once the child is settled into a routine and is on a stable insulin dose, I would suggest relaxing the number of tests done in order to improve compliance.

A regular pattern of diet is important. The child should be offered a diet high in complex carbohydrates, such as starch, which allow slow absorption and therefore slow rise in blood glucose. Refined sugars should be avoided. Fats should account for approximately 30% of the diet and should be predominantly polyunsaturated. A diet high in fibre will reduce the rise in blood glucose and also cholesterol. Essentially, the diabetic child should have a normal healthy diet; rigid rules are not helpful, since this encourages poor compliance. However, some families will find it helpful to be given a guide to the actual amount of carbohydrate that the child may eat at meal times and snacks. The carbohydrate exchange system, where 1 exchange is equivalent to 10 g of carbohydrate is then useful. Sample meal plans explained by the dietician are also valuable. A sensible approach to occasional treats should be maintained.

Exercise should be encouraged and the child should be able to continue his/her usual activities. Additional snacks should be taken if prolonged exercise is undertaken.

It is important not to burden the family with too much information about diabetes mellitus and the long-term complications on the first admission. The diagnosis and the short-term implications are alarming enough. However, it is important that they are told about hypoglycaemia, both how to recognise the symptoms and what to do when they occur, before discharge. I would also remind them that the insulin should not be stopped if the child is unwell and not eating, since this might cause ketoacidosis.

It is essential that the diabetic child is followed closely in the first few months to check progress and offer support. Where possible, a diabetic liaison nurse should be involved.

Perioperative diabetic management

Q. You are asked by the surgical team to oversee the diabetic management of a known insulin-dependent diabetic due to have (a) an orchidopexy and (b) major bowel surgery. What advice would you give?

Minor surgery

The child requires admission the night prior to surgery and should have his normal evening dose of insulin, but be starved from 3 am. He should then have 50% of his normal morning insulin dosage at 8 am on the day of surgery if a morning list but no breakfast. He needs to start an i.v. infusion of 10% dextrose at a maintenance dose at this time. It is important that he is first on the operating list and postoperatively he should be given lunch or high sugar drinks as tolerated. The i.v. dextrose infusion can be stopped when the patient is drinking adequately and he can be given his normal evening insulin dosage. Monitoring of the BM stix is carried out regularly, the frequency dependant upon stability of his blood sugar.

Major surgery

The child needs admission 1–2 days prior to surgery to monitor control. As before he needs to have his normal evening dose of insulin on the day before surgery. At 8 am the following day he should have an i.v. infusion of 10% dextrose with 1 g of KCl per 500 ml running in as maintenance. An i.v. insulin infusion should also be running concomitantly at a rate dependent on the hourly BM stix measurement. Postoperatively, the i.v. infusions must continue until the child is drinking and eating.

Height

Q. Why are boys taller than girls after puberty?

The average height of an adult female in the UK is 5 feet 4 inches (162 cm), whereas the average male is 5 feet 9 inches (175 cm). Up until around the age of 11, male and female heights are equal (both 142 cm as the 50th centile at age 11 on the Castlemead charts). At this age about 50% of girls will have breast stage 3 development and will be well into puberty, whereas only a few per cent of boys will be showing any evidence of early puberty. Between the ages of 11 and 14, girls on average are taller, but after age of 14 the boys overtake and ultimately are 5 inches taller.

The timing and intensity of the adolescent growth spurt is responsible for the size difference between adult men and women. The onset of this spurt is probably genetically controlled although its intensity and duration probably depend on hormonal factors. On average, boys enter the growth spurt 2 years later than girls. During this 2-year period, boys continue to grow at about 5 cm/year, the average height velocity of a child of either sex, just prior to entering the growth spurt. The girls on the other hand are shooting up at about 8 cm/year at this time. By the time they reach 14 years, the girls will have done most of their growing and the epiphyseal growth plates of the long bones will be fusing. At 14 years, the boys are at the peak of their height velocity, growing now at 8 cm/year. Therefore, because the boys enter this period of rapid growth 2 years later, they will have at least 10 cm extra growth before entering puberty. Epiphyseal fusion results from the action of hormones activated at puberty, and so if a child enters puberty earlier, they will stop growing sooner (in precocious puberty, the children are initially taller, but ultimately short). Complete fusion of the epiphyseal plates occurs at round 16–18 years in girls and 18–21 years in boys. Fusion occurs under the influence of high levels of oestrogens in women and testosterone in men.

Short stature

Q1. A 12-year-old girl is referred to the clinic after a school medical because of concern about short stature. How would you assess her?

The causes of short stature may be divided into four broad categories:

1. Familial
2. Constitutional delay of growth
3. Chronic systemic disorders
4. Endocrine abnormalities

I would try to establish which of these is the case for this girl by taking a history. I would record the birthweight and any known illnesses. I would ask when it was first noted that she was small for her age. I would also ask whether her parents had been small at her age or gone into puberty later than their friends.

On examination, I would accurately measure her height and weight. I would plot these on a standard growth chart, along with any other known previous measurements. I would check for signs of any chronic illnesses, e.g. heart murmurs suggestive of congenital heart disease; deformities of the chest suggestive of asthma; pallor, hypertension and nail changes suggestive of chronic renal failure; and finger clubbing and mouth ulcers suggestive of inflammatory bowel disease.

I would assess whether the girl was showing any signs of early puberty. I would also look for dysmorphic features, such as the triangular facies and clinodactyly of Silver-Russell syndrome or the shield chest, webbed neck and increased carrying angle of Turner's syndrome.

Ideally, I would measure the height of both parents. If unavailable, I would ask how tall they were. From these measurements, I would calculate the mid-parental height and centile. I would expect most children to reach a height at full growth within 8 cm of the mid-parental height centile. Of course, it is important to be sure that the parents do not also have a growth disorder, e.g. skeletal dysplasia or pseudohypoparathyroidism.

If the girl is significantly short, I would do a few baseline investigations on the first visit. If there is any history suggestive of a chronic illness, I would investigate as appropriate. If no abnormalities are detected in a previously well child, I would ask for an X-ray of the left wrist to check the bone age. If bone age is delayed, as it is with most causes of short stature, there is further potential for growth. I would check the karyotype of this girl, since the signs of Turner's syndrome are not always obvious, especially in the mosaic form. I would also check thyroid function, although there would usually be other signs of hypothyroidism at this age.

Unless there is an obvious abnormality, I would not investigate the girl further at this stage. I would arrange to see her in clinic several times over a period of a year and plot accurate height and weight measurements on these occasions. In this way, it is possible to calculate height velocity, which is a more specific measurement of growth. It would also be possible to assess development of puberty.

If the girl has a low height velocity and is not 'on target' to meet the expected growth potential according to mid-parental height, I would consider further investigation. It may be appropriate to perform a growth hormone provocation test. I am used to using the clonidine stimulation test. Clonidine is an α-adrenergic receptor stimulant and has been shown to facilitate growth hormone release. If the girl is not yet well established in puberty, I would want to prime her with oestrogens for 3 days prior to the test. Then she should be brought in to hospital for the day. After giving the clonidine orally, blood tests are taken at 30 minute intervals. The peak measurement of growth hormone should be at 90–120 minutes. The side-effects of clonidine are drowsiness, nausea and hypotension and the girl should be observed for these during and after the test before being allowed home.

Q2. The girl is found to have Turner's syndrome. How would you treat her?

Girls with Turner's syndrome have a low growth rate from the age of about 5. There is no growth spurt at puberty due to the absence of oestrogens. For this reason, the mean final height is approximately 140 cm, compared with an average mean height of 165 cm in normal girls. This can cause significant distress.

The cause of poor growth in Turner's syndrome is unclear, but some have true growth hormone deficiency. For this reason, I would perform a clonidine stimulation test. There may be only partial growth hormone deficiency. It has been shown that giving growth hormone to girls with Turner's syndrome improves growth over a period of 2 years. The long-term growth is not yet established.

The use of anabolic androgenic steroids also improves growth. The addition of low-dose oestrogens should also enhance growth. It is important to induce puberty at the age of about 13 in order to keep the patient in line with the progress of her peer group.

A knemometer

Q. Have you heard of a knemometer?

A knemometer is an electronic device for precisely and reproducibly measuring growth rate in children aged 5 years or more, over short periods of time. This usually means over days or weeks and for measurements of growth over longer periods it has nothing to offer over more conventional methods.

The child sits in an adjustable chair with his or her foot positioned flat on a template so a right angle is formed at the knee. The lower part of the leg is moved from side to side so that a low-friction measuring plateau placed on top of the knee accurately measures the maximum displacement from the foot template to within 0.1 mm. It has been shown that changes in the lower part of the lower limb are a good representation of true bone growth.

The knemometer is generally used as a research tool to measure the effects of diseases or treatments on growth. The knemometer demonstrates that growth at this level of accuracy is a non-linear, irregular process which proceeds as a series of mini growth spurts and lulls which are sensitive to intercurrent illness.

Constitutional delay in puberty

Q1. What is constitutional delay in growth and puberty?

Constitutional delay in growth and puberty (CDGP) is defined as delay of growth in otherwise healthy adolescents, with relatively reduced stature for chronological age, but generally appropriate for bone age, and delayed pubertal development. Since growth potential is related to the degree of epiphyseal maturation, the delay in bone age permits a final stature within the normal range. In other words, the height prognosis for these children is appropriate for their parental centiles.

There is a familial tendency to constitutional delay in growth and puberty. It tends to affect more boys than girls. This is probably due to the difference in sensitivity to gonadotrophin releasing hormone between the sexes. Girls produce gonadotrophins in response to small amounts of gonadotrophin releasing hormone, which explains why precocious puberty is more common in girls. Boys are much less sensitive to gonadotrophin releasing hormone and therefore puberty is normally later in adolescence. In CDGP the amount of gonadotrophin releasing hormone required to trigger gonadotrophin release is reached even later.

Constitutional delay in growth and puberty is a common cause of growth delay and is probably an extreme of the normal range of growth patterns. Extensive investigation is unnecessary and the biochemical results may be misleading; therefore, the diagnosis should be made on anthropometric evidence. The child has relatively short spinal length compared to leg length. If a child has extreme short stature and decelerating growth, the diagnosis is less likely to be CDGP and further investigation is warranted.

Q2. Should these children be treated?

Although constitutional delay in growth and puberty seems to be a physiological variant of normal, it can cause enormous anxiety to the affected individual. Peer group pressure is very influential during puberty and comparison to others is then distressing. Boys are more commonly affected and tend to suffer more due to social pressures. The boy may be bullied and behaviour may become deviant, leading to truancy, shoplifting and vandalism. School performance will be affected and therefore future careers. Treatment allows the boy to keep pace with his peers. It has been shown that, although distressed during adolescence, most patients do not continue to have low self-esteem in adult life.

Adults who have had untreated CDGP seem to be at higher risk of osteoporosis. Skeletal disproportion, i.e. relatively short spine compared to leg length, also persists.

For these reasons, it seems sensible to treat these adolescents if a safe and effective treatment is available.

Q3. What treatments are available to these adolescents?

Treatments used in constitutional delay in growth and puberty are based on normal physiology of growth. Growth hormone and sex steroids are both required for normal growth. Changes in growth velocity are secondary to the pulse amplitude of growth hormone, mainly secreted at night. Sex steroids temporarily increase growth hormone secretion.

Treatment options include:

1. *Anabolic steroids*, e.g. oxandralone. These work by increasing growth hormone secretion. A low-dose daily regimen will induce a growth spurt which continues once the steriods are stopped. They induce normal advancement in secondary sexual characteristics and have been shown to double the height velocity. Previously, they were used in high doses but this caused inappropriate advancement of bone age and therefore lower than predicted final height. This is not a problem at low dosage. Final height is not improved, but accelerated.
2. *Testosterone*. This induces secondary sexual characteristics, but the levels of hormone fluctuate whether given orally or by deep i.m. depot injection. Testosterone should be given for a period of 3 months to allow a sustained growth spurt. (Oestrogen will have the same effect in girls.) Human chorionic gonadotrophin is a more physiological method of increasing sex hormones. However, it has to be given by injection 3 times a week to produce sustained levels. Sex steroids can be used when inadequate sexual development is the main complaint.
3. *Growth hormone*. This has been used mainly in growth hormone deficient children. It has, however, been shown to increase height velocity in boys with constitutional delay if given in high doses for a long period of time. It should then improve final height prognosis, since epiphyseal maturation is not advanced.

Precocious puberty

Q. A mother brings her 5-year-old daughter to clinic concerned that she has started pubertal development. How would you approach her management?

I would want to discover which signs of puberty have developed and in which order they became obvious. Normal pubertal development (with the signs of breast development, then pubic hair and finally menarche) occurring at an early age is said to show consonance. These girls have early activation of the hypothalamic–pituitary–gonadal axis. If there is lack of consonance, it implies sex hormone production independent of the hypothalamus and is otherwise known as pseudopuberty.

Many cases of precocious puberty in girls are *constitutional*. These children are likely to have breast enlargement at presentation, then progress to normal puberty. Although there is usually no structural cause to trigger puberty, small hamartomas in the region of the hypothalamus may activate gonadotrophin releasing hormone. These girls can expect a normal reproductive life, but may have relatively short stature due to early epiphyseal fusion. I would ask about other signs of hypothalamic disturbance, such as polydipsia, polyuria, obesity and sleep problems. It may be due to cerebral tumours, hydrocephalus, e.g. late presentation of aqueduct stenosis, trauma and central nervous system infection, e.g. tuberculous meningitis. Once the diagnosis is clarified, a treatment plan can be drawn up.

Other causes of true precocious puberty include severe hypothyroidism, neurofibromatosis and the McCune-Albright syndrome. These diagnoses should be apparent on clinical examination. In the case of *hypothyroidism* the child may be obese and short with dry skin, coarse facial features and slow heart rate. I would look for the fibromatous skin lesions and café-au-lait patches of *neurofibromatosis* and ask about similar lesions in other family members. Pigmented skin lesions may also be present in *McCune Albright syndrome*, when bony sclerotic lesions may also accompany hormonal imbalance.

Pseudopuberty, where consonance is lacking, may be due to *ingestion of sex hormones* in this child. I would ask whether she could have found oral contraceptive pills in the house, since this is a cause of sexual development, especially vaginal bleeding, which requires no further investigation and would be of great reassurance to the parents.

Pseudopuberty may be due to *ovarian tumours*. In these cases the tumour may be palpable on abdominal examination by the time endocrine effects are apparent. The tumour is most frequently of the granulosa theca cell type and is therefore usually benign.

Isolated *premature thelarche* occurs in young girls and further investigation may be unnecessary if puberty proceeds no further on review. Breast enlargement in these girls usually regresses in 3–4 years.

I would measure and plot the height and weight on centile charts when the girl is brought to clinic. Careful assessment of the stage of puberty should be made. If vaginal bleeding is the only symptom, I would want to exclude the possibility of a foreign body.

My initial investigations would include:

1. *Bone age* — which will be advanced in true precocious puberty, but delayed in hypothyroidism.
2. *Skull X-ray* — may show signs of raised intracranial pressure or calcification.
3. *Oestrogen levels* — will be increased in most cases, but are likely to be much higher in an oestrogen-secreting tumour.
4. *Androgen levels and 17-hydroxyprogesterone* — high if pubic hair and rapid growth are a prominent feature.
5. *Serum gonadotrophins* — will be high in a central cause, but reduced in a secreting ovarian tumour or if exogenous hormones have been taken.
6. *Pelvic ultrasound* — simple and non-invasive and excludes ovarian masses.
7. *Gonadotrophin releasing hormone stimulation test* — there will be an increased response in true precocious puberty.

Finally, I would consider CT scan or MRI of the head if I am concerned that intracranial pathology might account for the advanced development.

I feel it is important to exclude serious pathology in a girl of 5 since intervention will reduce anxiety and improve the child's final height. In an older girl, my investigations would be more limited, since constitutional puberty would be the most likely cause.

Nephrotic syndrome

Q. What can you tell me about nephrotic syndrome?

Nephrotic syndrome is defined as:

1. Hypoalbuminaemia — serum albumin <25 mg/l
2. Proteinuria — >40 mg/h/m^2
3. Oedema

In childhood the majority of cases have three histological changes:

1. Minimal change glomerulonephritis   85%
2. Focal segmental glomerulosclerosis   10%
3. Mesangiocapillary glomerulonephritis   5%

but classification is more usually divided, not into histological pattern, but responsiveness to oral steroids, because in the majority of cases, no renal biopsy is performed.

a) *Steroid-resistant nephrotic syndrome*, i.e. not responding (persistence of proteinuria) with 28 days of oral prednisolone (60 mg/m^2/day up to a maximum of 80 mg/day). These can be predicted to a certain extent by age of onset (<6 months or >12 years), presence of gross haematuria (in the absence of infection) and persistent microscopic haematuria if associated with hypertension and/or low plasma C3. These infants/children should undergo renal biopsy at the outset and be under the full time care of a paediatric nephrologist.

b) *Steroid-sensitive nephrotic syndrome*. This is of unknown aetiology, although loss of charge selectivity in the glomerular basement membrane due to cationic protein production has been put forward as the cause of albumin leak. It usually occurs in the 2–6 year olds with a ratio of 2 : 1 male to female and very often is preceded by an upper respiratory tract infection.

Investigation

— urine microscopy and culture; early morning urine protein/creatinine ratio (>200 mg/mmol in nephrotic syndrome); NB ~ 30% have microscopic haematuria at presentation
— blood serum U & Es, albumin, creatinine FBC and haematocrit. Hepatitis B surface antigen, ?lipids/cholesterol, ?ASOT, C3, C4, ANF

Management

— blood pressure, height and weight on admission

— avoidance of bed rest, unless grossly oedematous
— no added salt diet, i.e. no added salt to food at the table
— (Various diets have been advocated in the past but have been discounted)
— fluid restriction: avoidance of excessive fluid intake rather than restriction, unless grossly oedematous.
— oral penicillin: at presentation until the oedema has settled to prevent septicaemia and peritonitis from *Streptococcus pneumoniae* particularly (the risk occurs because of loss of opsonins and immunoglobulins in the urine)
— treatment of hypovolaemia if present with 20 ml/kg PPF followed by salt poor albumin 1 g/kg body weight as a 20% solution over 1–2 hours with frusemide cover
— treatment of hypertension:
    i) secondary to hypervolaemia
    ii) secondary to vasoconstrictive response to hypovolaemia. Atenolol (0.5–1 mg/kg) o.d. and/or nifedipine (0.25–2 mg/kg/day divided by 2)
— steroids
    i) Initial episode. Prednisolone 60 mg/kg/m^2/day (maximum 80 mg/day) until remission, followed by 40 mg/kg/m^2 (maximum 60 mg/day) on alternate days for 4 weeks
    ii) First two relapses. Prednisolone 60 mg/m^2/day (maximum 80 mg/day) until remission, followed by 40 mg/m^2/day (maximum 60 mg/day) on alternate days for 4 weeks
    iii) Frequent relapses. Maintenance prednisolone 0.1–0.5 mg/kg alternate days for 3–6 months, then reduce
    iv) Relapse on prednisolone >0.5 mg/kg/alternate days. Levamisole 2.5 mg/kg alternate days for 4–12 months
    v) Relapse on prednisolone >0.5 mg/kg/alternate days and steroid side-effects or risk factors or relapse on steroids >1.0 mg/kg alternate days. Cyclophosphamide 3 mg/kg/day for 8 weeks
    vi) Post-cyclophosphamide relapses. As ii) and iii) above
    vii) Relapse on prednisolone >0.5 mg/kg/alternate days. Cyclosporin 5 mg/kg/day for 1 year
    viii) Relapse on cyclosporin?
NB. Relapse = 3+ proteinuria for 3 days or 2+ proteinuria for 10 days.
— Vaccinations. Immunise once off daily steroids for 3 months. Dead vaccines when in remission. Varicella zoster immunoglubin should be given if on high-dose steroids/alkylating agents, on exposure to chickenpox and acyclovir immediately if chickenpox occurs. ?The value of polyvalent pneumococcal vaccination

Prognosis
There are no predictors for this, but at least 60% and probably >75% will relapse. Parents should test the urine every morning for proteinuria and if 3+ for 3 consecutive days or 2+ for 10 consecutive days, they should seek medical advice.

Children on long-term steroids should be assessed regularly for growth, blood pressure measurement and once yearly for the development of subcapsular cataracts.

Unanswered questions about nephrotic syndrome

1. Dosage and duration of high-dose steroids. German data suggests that 60 mg/m^2/day for 6 weeks followed by 40 mg/m^2/alternate days for a further 6 weeks may reduce the risk of relapse.
2. The use of lipid-lowering agents. Hyperlipidaemia is usually a transient state, but if prolonged, serum lipid lowering agents, e.g. simvastatin may be justified.
3. The value of pneumovax administration.
4. The effectiveness of other immunosuppressant agents in chronic relapsing nephrotic syndrome if conventional treatments are not successful.

Erythropoietin

Q1. Tell me about erythropoietin.

Erythropoietin is a glycoprotein hormone produced by the combination of renal produced factor (probably from the juxtaglomerular cells and glomeruli — this being one of the endocrine functions of the kidney) and a plasma globulin. Its production is stimulated in response to anaemia or when erythrocytes are unable to liberate oxygen for other reasons and it has a short circulating half-life of 4–12 hours. Erythropoietin is the main stimulus for erythropoiesis in the body which it does by increasing erythropoietic stem cells, stimulating haemoglobin synthesis and decreasing the maturation time of precursors. The increase in circulating red cells therefore takes 2–3 days to appear. The anatomical expansion of bone marrow can be severe in chronic anaemias and explains, for example, the frontal bossing, etc. seen in β-thalassaemia.

Loss of erythropoietin is the reason for the normocytic normochromic anaemia of chronic renal failure and excess of erythropoietin is the mechanism for the polycythaemia found in some patients with polycystic renal disease or renal cysts.

Q2. Do you know anything about clinical applications of erythropoietin?

Manufactured erythropoietin is now available as a result of recombinant DNA technology. Its major application is in the treatment of anaemia of end-stage chronic renal failure in patients maintained on haemodialysis, where the need for repeated blood transfusions can be abolished. Clinical studies have confirmed its effectiveness and consistently good results have been obtained not only in the correction of anaemia but also in quality of life, improved exercise tolerance and cardiorespiratory function.

It is administered 3 times weekly at body-weight dependant doses by i.v. injection over 2–3 minutes. The haemoglobin response is monitored and doses may be slowly increased. Sometimes iron or vitamin supplements are required with erythropoietin therapy. The more serious adverse effects of erythropoietin relate to thrombosis of vascular access sites, clotting in the dialyser, hyperkalaemia, hypertension and seizures. Minor side-effects include viraemia-like symptoms, headache and rashes. Its major limiting factor is its cost.

It is currently being evaluated in the management of anaemia in premature infants (Halperin et al 1990, Shannon et al 1992) and this may prove to be a promising new application.

REFERENCES

Halperin D S et al 1990 Effects of recombinant human erythropoietin in infants with the anaemia of
    prematurity: a pilot study. J Pediatr 116: 779–786
Shannon K M et al 1992 Enhancement of erythropoiesis by recombinant human erythropoietin in
    low birth weight infants: a pilot study. J Pediatr 120: 586-592

Haemolytic uraemic syndrome

Q. What can you tell me about the pathogenesis of the haemolytic uraemic syndrome?

Haemolytic uraemic syndrome is characterised by the triad of microangiopathic haemolytic anaemia, thrombocytopaenia and renal failure. The exact pathogenesis is uncertain, but it may be the end result of different initiating agents. This may explain the two distinct clinical types.

1. The *epidemic* variety is more common and tends to affect infants and young children during the summer months. There is usually a prodromal illness of diarrhoea. Generally, the prognosis is good with supportive management. Hypertension and neurological involvement are rare. Siblings may develop the disorder within days of one another.

2. The *sporadic* variety is less common and affects older children at any time of year. It is sometimes preceded by a mild respiratory illness. The prognosis is much worse for renal function and there may be severe hypertension. Neurological involvement is common. If siblings develop the same disorder, it tends to be a year or more apart, suggesting that there is no infective cause, but may be a genetic predisposition.

The epidemic nature of the most common type of haemolytic uraemic syndrome suggests that there is an infective cause. A similar syndrome has been found in Bangladeshi children following Shigella infection, however this organism has not been isolated in other children. A variety of other organisms had been implicated, but none had been consistently isolated until reports of an association with verotoxin-producing *Escherichia coli* (serotype 0157:H7) in 1983. The verotoxin is similar in structure to the Shigella toxin. It is unknown how the toxin produces the syndrome, but it has been suggested that it may be directly toxic to the renal endothelial cell.

The pathological changes in the kidney also suggest that there are two distinct types of haemolytic uraemic syndrome. The epidemic variety tends to be associated with predominantly glomerular involvement, with thrombotic microangiopathy, while the sporadic variety tends to be associated with predominantly arteriolar involvement. The importance of these different histopathological patterns is uncertain, but it may be related to the site of action of the toxin.

It is the thrombotic occlusion of small blood vessels which causes the microangiopathic disorder. It had been suggested that haemolytic uraemic syndrome might be caused by the activation of the coagulation pathway, presumably by the infective agent. However, clotting studies are usually only mildly abnormal with normal fibrinogen turnover and trials of anti-coagulation have proved ineffective in the treatment of the disorder.

Platelet aggregation is increased in some cases, which may explain the thrombosis in small blood vessels. There may be an additional factor which induces platelet aggregation in the plasma of patients with haemolytic uraemic syndrome. Alternatively, there may be deficiency of a factor which normally inhibits platelet aggregation. Certainly, adding normal plasma to a patient's plasma in vitro seems to inhibit aggregation.

Prostaglandins are involved in platelet aggregation. Prostacyclin is produced from arachidonic acid in the endothelial cell and is a powerful inhibitor of platelet aggregation. Thromboxane is metabolised from arachidonic acid in the platelet and is a platelet aggregating agent. Prostacyclin activity has been shown to be reduced in the plasma of patients with the sporadic form of the disease. However, this is not a consistent finding and infusions of prostacyclin or fresh plasma in the treatment of haemolytic uraemic syndrome have had variable success.

In summary, the pathogenesis of haemolytic uraemic syndrome is unknown, but it may be related to the effect of a toxin on renal endothelium in the epidemic variety and is likely to be due to an imbalance in platelet aggregation factors in the sporadic variety.

REFERENCE

Levin M, Barratt T M 1984 Haemolytic uraemic syndrome. Arch Dis Child 59: 397–400

Urinary tract infection

Q1. How would you investigate urinary tract infections in children?

Symptomatic urinary tract infections (UTIs) occur in ~3% of girls and 1% of boys during childhood. In the majority it is an isolated infection with no predisposing factors and no long-term sequelae. However, investigation is justified in all cases if only to prevent a small proportion of these children developing end-stage renal failure.

Investigation is dependent on *age* of the child at presentation. In all an appropriate collection of urine is necessary in order to make a diagnosis of UTI and this can very often be the most difficult part of the management. Undoubtedly, some children will undergo investigations for UTI, although in reality they never had an infection, due to this difficulty.

1. *In children under 1 year of age.*
Suprapubic aspiration (SPA) of urine is the gold standard method of urine collection, although unpleasant for infant and parent alike. If there is a high clinical suspicion of UTI, I would perform an SPA. Some advocate the use of ultrasound guidance to improve the success rate, although I have little experience of this. Urgent microscopy would show white cells ($50 \times 10^9/1$) and organisms ($>10^5$/ml) in UTI, provided antibiotics had not been given previously.

The use of 'clean catch' and bags for urine collection is less satisfactory, but may be warranted. Ideally I would collect at least two samples by these methods prior to starting antibiotics.

2. *In children aged 1–3 years.*
I would not undertake SPA in these children, but would rely on clean catch urines as far as possible. In the older child, mid-stream urine (MSU) collection may be practical.

3. *Children over 3 years of age.*
At least two MSUs prior to starting antibiotic therapy would be warranted. The use of catheter specimen of urine (SCU) collection can be justified occasionally, but it has the risk of introduction of bacteria into the bladder.

Once I have collected my sample(s) of urine and appropriate treatment has been implemented, subsequent investigation is again dependent on age. Broadly speaking:

1. *Neonates.*
A full septic screen including lumbar puncture is necessary, plus renal ultrasound scan during the hospital stay, followed by at least a micturating cystourethrogram (MCUG) at 4–6 weeks after discharge. Evidence of reflux, renal

cortical damage, pelvi-calyceal dilatation, etc. would require further investigation (e.g. DMSA, DTPA, cystoscopy).

2. *Under 2 year olds*.
Plain abdominal X-ray, renal USS and MCUG in all. In good hands, renal ultrasonography is excellent at detection of renal scarring. Some radiologists would suggest that the plain abdominal X-ray is an unnecessary exposure to radiation and all the information obtained could be achieved from ultrasonography alone.

3. *2–5 year olds*.
For these children renal USS may be sufficient, but if recurrent UTIs or abnormalities are picked up on the USS, an MCUG may be necessary, or other investigations.

4. *Over 5 year olds*.
For a child with their first UTI, I would carry out renal ultrasonography, although if any renal scarring had occured it may well have been many years previously.

In children under 2 years of age, I would give the child a 5-day course of antibiotics initially and continue with a night-time prophylactic dose until the renal USS and MCUG have been performed, the latter being carried out 4–6 weeks after the initial infection.

Q2. Tell me about other radiological tests for the investigation of UTI in childhood.

1. *DMSA scan* (99m Tc–dimercaptosuccinic acid scintigraphy). This is a superb test for looking at anatomical abnormalities of the kidneys, most notably renal scarring. DMSA is selectively taken up by the renal tubules and gamma radiation is emitted, with scars showing up as parenchymal filling defects on the scan. It must be borne in mind that it does not differentiate between acute and chronic scarring.
2. *DTPA scan* (99m Tc–diethylenetriamene pentaacetic acid scan). This is a functional test of the renal tract and is very useful in differentiating between simple dilatation (i.e. mega-ureter) and obstruction, causing dilatation (i.e. vesico-ureteric junction, pelvic-ureteric junction).
3. *51 Cr/EDTA scan*. A test used for glomerular filtration rate measurement that involves gamma emission measurement of blood at 2 and 4 hours post-injection of the radioactive label. This test allows measurement of differential function of the two kidneys.

Haematuria

Q1. How would you investigate a child that has haematuria?

The answer is dependent upon the likely cause of the haematuria. In the majority of cases, it will be microscopic and detected by diagnostic urinary dipsticks. These are exquisitely sensitive at picking up blood in urine and therefore positivity may not be indicative of disease. Contamination from menstrual blood or from the perineum will give a positive result, as will exercise. It is therefore important to re-check the urine and undertake urine microscopy and culture. Urine microscopy is very useful, not only to confirm the presence of RBCs but also to look at morphology of the red cells (lower urinary tract blood tends to have well preserved red cells, whereas upper renal tract bleeding results in dysmorphic cells). Microscopy can also reveal the presence of crystals, white cells, organisms and casts.

Causes of haematuria include the following broad categories:

1. Urinary tract infection (10^5 organisms/ml and $10^5/1$ white cells)
2. Nephritis   — Henoch-Schönlein purpura (60% have haematuria at presentation)
   — Post-infectious glomerulonephritis
   — IgA nephropathy
   — Alport's syndrome
   — Nephrotic syndrome (~30% have haematuria at presentation)
3. Stones
4. Trauma
5. Haematological   — Coagulopathies: HUS, ITP
   — Sickle cell disease
6. Anatomical causes — Polycystic/multicystic kidneys
   — Tumours
7. Munchausen syndrome by proxy
8. Miscellaneous   — Drugs: cyclophosphamide, aspirin
   — Recurrent benign haematuria (the diagnosis of exclusion)

Of all the above causes UTI, HSP, HUS, post-infectious glomerulonephritis and recurrent benign haematuria account for the majority. History, examination and urinalysis will direct one to a likely cause.

Pertinent points in the history are:

1. Urinary tract symptoms: dysuria, frequency, urgency
2. Previous history of haematuria

3. History of trauma
4. History of preceding illness, i.e. URTI, diarrhoea
5. Family history of deafness.

Examination

1. Blood pressure measurement.
2. Presence of peripheral oedema/ascites.
3. Presence of abdominal mass.
4. Skin changes, i.e. vasculitic rash, purpura.

Investigation

1. Urine culture — indicated in all cases of haematuria.
2. Routine biochemistry — creatinine, calcium, albumin.
3. Haematology — FBC + coagulation studies.
4. Renal ultrasound scan.
5. Other blood tests — if a nephritic picture, consider ANF, ASOT, complement, hepatitis B surface antigen.
6. Renal biopsy — this should be performed only in specialist tertiary centres and only as a third-line investigation. Indications would include suggestive nephritis (haematuria, oedema and hypertension), persistent abnormal renal function or persistent unexplained haematuria.
7. Other investigations:
   — Radionucleotide scans
   — Urine calcium/creatinine ratio
   — Intravenous pyelogram
   — Cystoscopy
   — Urine microscopy of relatives

Treatment and prognosis is dependent upon cause.

REFERENCE

Rath B, Turner C, Hartley B, Chantler C 1991 Evaluation of light microscopy to localise the site of haematuria. Arch Dis Child 66: 338–340

Oncology, haematology and rheumatology

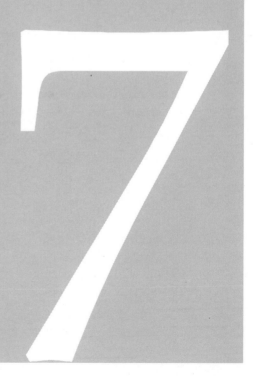

7

Complications of chemotherapy

Q. What are the problems of chemotherapy in the treatment of childhood cancers?

I would like to divide this question up into three broad sections:

1. General side-effects of the chemotherapeutic agents
2. Specific and idiosyncratic side-effects of individual drugs
3. Long-term sequelae of treatment

1. *General side-effects.*

The majority of childhood cancers today are treated with nationally coordinated intensive combination chemotherapy protocols that are greatly improving long-term remission rates. All the cytotoxic agents have adverse effects and many of these can be predicted since tumour cells are not selectively destroyed. Rapidly proliferating cells such as those in the bone marrow, gastrointestinal tract, oral mucosa and hair follicles are also affected, resulting in adverse and often dose-limiting toxicity. The severity of these side-effects is dependent on dose and frequency of administration and recovery time allowed between treatment courses.

Most agents used result in nausea and vomiting, marrow suppression (bleomycin being an exception, but it is rarely used in childhood), alopecia and stomatitis.

Very often nausea and vomiting can be the most feared problem a child faces during his/her chemotherapy. It is therefore important to start anti-emetic measures early and continue them throughout the period of rapid cell turnover. Agents used include metoclopramide, lorazepam, nabilone (a synthetic cannabinoid) and ondansetron — this is a selective 5-HT$_3$ receptor antagonist, used extensively in paediatric oncology because of its efficacy and minimal side-effects.

At presentation children with cancer may be neutropenic, anaemic and thrombocytopenia due to bone marrow involvement. Virtually all agents used will result in further damage to the stem cells. Neutropaenia and thrombocytopaenia are the major problems of this damage which can lead to their own potentially fatal sequelae.

Alopecia is a distressing side-effect of treatment that if dealt with appropriately and sensitively should cause little problem to patient or family.

2. *Specific side-effects*

a) *Cardiotoxicity*. Most notably cardiotoxic are the anthracyclines doxorubicin and daunorubicin. This frequently fatal dose-related side-effect has no treatment other than transplantation and is difficult to detect (except by endomyocardial biopsy) until established damage has occurred. Monitoring with echocardiography is advised.

b) *Pulmonary toxicity*. Bleomycin is the major culprit with lung damage occurring in 10% of patients and death in 1–2%. Again damage is dose related.

c) *Neurotoxicity*. Vincristine, an alkaloid agent, most commonly produces a mixed distal sensorimotor neuropathy with long-term use. Initially sensory changes with paraesthesia progresses to loss of deep tendon reflexes and is an indication to stop vincristine administration as severe incoordination and seizures may develop. Vincristine also has an effect on autonomic function commonly resulting in troublesome constipation and even paralytic ileus.

d) *Urological toxicity*. Many cytotoxics are excreted by the kidneys and it is therefore important to check renal function prior to initiating a course of chemotherapy. Pre-, peri- and post-hydration plus alkalinisation of the urine can prevent or minimise cytotoxic deposition and consequent damage to the renal tubules. Methotrexate, cisplatin ifosphamide and carboplatin are all nephrotoxic. Dose adjustment in renal impairment is mandatory.

    The alkylating agents cyclophosphamide and ifosphamide can cause haemorrhagic cystitis, having a cumulative and dose-related effect. Acrolein, one of the breakdown products, is the causative substance. Adequate hydration and mesna administration lessens this damage.

I have mentioned only the more common and well known side-effects of agents used widely in paediatric oncology. However, the agents can have an effect on other systems including skin, bones and joints, electrolytes, liver, etc. and each agent can affect more than one system, e.g. cyclophosphamide and cardiotoxicity, sterility and pulmonary toxicity.

3. *Long-term effects.*

With almost 60% of children treated for cancer now acheiving long-term survival, long-term side-effects take on heightened importance. Initial chemotherapy courses may be of short duration, but follow-up is continued long term. For children who relapse or who are on prolonged chemotherapy courses, there will be long periods of time in hospital and concomitant time away from siblings, peers, friends and very importantly school. During this time the whole dynamics of the family may change considerably from engendering stability as the family rallies round to support or obversely, disruption if one family member is unable to cope with the inevitable change in lifestyle. Sibling rivalry may cause a great deal of antagonism as another child loses the once equal share of parental attention. Financially the family may be disadvantaged because of frequent travel between home and hospital, and one or both parents may have to give up their employment to take up the full time job of looking after the patient.

Long-term sequelae of the chemotherapy that can be difficult to broach with the patient include:

a) Infertility — more a problem for boys than girls and compounded by radiotherapy. In adolescents and young adults, sperm cryopreservation is justifiable.

b) Late recurrence — with 5-year long-term remission most would be considered 'cured' of the cancer but relapse can occur after this time.

c) Secondary neoplasia — occuring in between 1 and 4% of childhood patients. The increased risk is dependent very much on the nature of the cancer, the chemotherapy and whether or not radiotherapy was used.

Management of neutropaenia

Q. How would you manage a leukaemic child with chemotherapy-induced neutropaenia?

Neutropaenia in a child with leukaemia may be secondary to bone marrow infiltration and suppression by cytotoxic agents. The child is at risk from bacterial and fungal infection when the neutrophil count is $<1.0 \times 10^9/1$. Life-threatening infections are more likely to occur at neutrophil counts of $0.2 \times 10^9/1$. It should be remembered that these children also have lymphopaenia and impaired immunoglobulin production secondary to treatment protocols. This is particularly true in children who have undergone bone marrow transplantation. Therefore, host mechanisms are greatly reduced and the child should be protected from infection where possible.

The timing of the neutropaenia can usually be predicted from the chemotherapeutic agents used and preventative measures should be taken. The pathogens which most frequently cause infection are the patient's normal flora: skin flora, such as *Staphylococcus aureus* and *epidermidis*, and bowel flora, such as coliforms, pseudomonas and klebsiella.

The risk of infection by organisms which frequent the mouth can be reduced by using mouthwashes such as 0.1% hibitane. If mouth ulcers develop, difflam is useful since it is antibacterial and has some local anaesthetic properties. Regular use of an oral anti-fungal agent, such as nystatin, will reduce the frequency of candida infection of the mucous membranes. This in turn will reduce the incidence of systemic candida infection, due to reduced invasion of oral organisms. However, nystatin is not absorbed and is therefore not completely protective against systemic infection. For those at particularly high risk of infection, e.g. after bone marrow transplantation, an oral agent such as ketoconazole or fluconazole might be more effective. Vigorous tooth brushing should be avoided, since this may provide the organisms with a port of entry.

Hand washing by staff and relatives should be meticulous. This is particularly important when taking blood, especially from central venous lines, when sterile gloves should be worn. Rectal examination and the use of suppositories should be avoided during neutropaenia, since this may also allow gut flora to become invasive.

The child with neutropaenia should be watched carefully for signs of infection. If the child has a white cell count of <1, there must be a low threshold for treatment with intravenous antibiotics. A child who is unwell with non-specific symptoms or is peripherally shut down, or has a fever of 38°C or more on two separate occasions at hourly intervals, should be screened for infection. This should include surface and throat swabs, blood and urine cultures. A chest X-ray is also necessary. Swabs from the entry site and central blood cultures should be included in those with a central venous line. Broad-spectrum antibiotics are then started immediately without waiting for culture results. I am used to using the combination of a penicillin and aminoglycoside, e.g. azlocillin and gentamicin, as a first line. This should cover the most likely organisms, including pseudomonas. If these antibiotics do not reduce the temperature and make the child feel better by 48 hours, I would consider changing the antibiotics. If nothing has been grown on culture (which is often the case), I would start a new-generation cephalosporin, e.g. cefotaxime or ceftazidime. If there is no improvement by a further 2 days, I would be suspicious of a systemic fungal infection and consider starting an anti-fungal agent, e.g. amphotericin. Amphotericin should be started at a low dose and it is important to check renal function. Hypokalaemia is a frequent problem.

Many of these infections are probably viral in origin and the child usually starts to feel better when the white cell count increases.

Bone marrow transplantation

Q. What are the indications for bone marrow transplantation in children?

Bone marrow transplantation is most commonly used in malignant disease. It should be considered in *acute myeloid leukaemia* (AML), particularly in high-risk groups. This will include those with a high white cell count at diagnosis; those with cytogenetic abnormalities such as monosomy 7 or 5 and those with a high blast count after 28 days of chemotherapy. For these children, bone marrow transplantation should be attempted as soon as the child is in remission, since relapse rate is high, and once relapse occurs prognosis is poor. For children in a low-risk group (such as those with a low white cell count at diagnosis; those with translocation of chromosome 8 and 21; and those with a low blast count after 28 days of treatment) the prognosis appears to be the same after a further course of chemotherapy or bone marrow transplantation. This is due to the mortality risk from the procedure itself.

When bone marrow transplantation is considered beneficial, a suitable donor needs to be found. Ideally this should be a histocompatibility locus antigen (HLA) identical donor. There is a 25% chance of a sibling being compatible. It is possible to use an unrelated but matched donor, but there is a higher rate of rejection.

The case for using bone marrow transplantation in *acute lymphoblastic leukaemia* (ALL) is less well defined. The prognosis for ALL in children is generally good, with 75% survival at 5 years. It may be used after relapse, when a second complete remission has been induced. The outcome is improved by 40% in the transplant group compared with standard treatment. There are certain groups with high risk factors where earlier transplantation can be considered. These include null cell or B cell leukaemia, children who present under the age of 1 year and those with a high white cell count at presentation.

Bone marrow transplantation is also considered in other malignant disorders with a poor prognosis, such as *Stage IV neuroblastoma*.

Other indications include:

— *acquired aplastic anaemia*
— *congenital bone marrow disorders*, e.g. congenital neutropaenia
— *immunodeficiency syndromes*, e.g. severe combined immunodeficiency
— *chronic granulomatous disease*
— *metabolic disorders*, e.g. mucopolysaccharidoses
— *haemoglobinopathies*, e.g. thalassaemia sickle cell anaemia

Bone marrow transplantation is still an experimental procedure for the rare metabolic disorders, but can be considered in those with a poor prognosis if a histocompatible family member is available. Obviously, the disorder must be excluded in the sibling donor.

Transplantation from an unmatched, related donor, such as a haplotype parent, can be considered in critical cases, such as infants with severe combined immunodeficiency. Rejection is less likely, as they are unable to mount a good immune response. It is particularly important to exclude infection prior to transplant in these children.

Bone marrow transplantation is not without risk and should only be considered in those children with haemoglobinopathy if they are transfusion dependant and have a histocompatible sibling. The child must have normal liver function tests to exclude iron overload. The mortality rate of bone marrow transplantation is lower in non-malignant disease and is curative, therefore it may be cost effective.

Care of the dying child

Q. How would you care for the terminally ill child?

The aim of palliative care is to give the child as good a quality of life as is possible in the final stages of a chronic illness. The child should be allowed to die peacefully and with dignity. Terminal care can be considered in two parts. *symptom relief* and *explanation and support*.

Pain is the most common unpleasant symptom experienced and should be treated aggressively. Initially, mild general discomfort can be treated with paracetamol, sometimes with the addition of non-steroidal anti-inflammatory drugs, particularly if bone pain is a problem. It is essential to give analgesia regularly, rather than on a 'as required' basis, since pain is much more difficult to control if it is recurrent. There should be no hesitation to use opiates if palliative care is considered to be appropriate. This can be given orally as tablets or elixir. Once a satisfactory dose has been found, it is possible to give slow-release morphine twice a day. 'Top up' analgesia, in the form of short-acting morphine can still be given. If the child is unable to take oral medication, an i.v. diamorphine infusion can be given if a central venous line is in place. Alternatively, diamorphine can be given by constant infusion subcutaneously. The child may feel sleepy on starting morphine, but this effect usually wears off in a few days. The parents should be reassured that morphine addiction is not a problem when used in this situation. The dose of morphine might need regular adjustment, since tolerance does occur.

Persistent pain is sometimes a problem. If the pain is localised, it may be possible to reduce it using a nerve block. It should be remembered that intractable pain may be due to psychological distress and may be relieved by discussion of the underlying worries.

Nausea and vomiting may be a problem, either due to the disease itself or the analgesia. Regular anti-emetics, such as metoclopramide, are usually effective. The child on a diamorphine infusion may get relief from the addition of an anti-emetic, such as cyclizine.

Constipation can be expected to occur in the majority of terminally ill patients, due to general debility, poor fluid intake and the use of opiates. This should be avoided by the early introduction of a gentle laxative, such as lactulose.

Other symptoms might include: pruritis — which may be helped by the addition of an anti-histamine; urinary retention — which sometimes requires catheterisation; bleeding — if the platelet count is low due to the primary disease. Platelet transfusion can be given if this becomes a distressing symptom.

The *psychological care* of the terminally ill child must centre around the whole family. Honesty should be encouraged. Even very young children will be aware that something is seriously wrong and will be frightened if no-one can explain what is happening to them. Fear of death is often less for children than for adults, who have different expectations. A child may already have developed their own ideas about death, from the experience of losing a pet or older relative. They may be helped by talking about what happens after they die. Some children may wish to make a will to divide their possessions amongst family and friends. Others may want to plan music or readings for their funeral.

Both the parents and child may ask exactly how the child will die and will be relieved if it is explained that most children die peacefully when symptomatic relief is maximised.

It is important to involve the siblings where appropriate, as they may feel neglected if not given proper explanations. Resentment of the ill child may then occur. As far as possible, the family routine should be maintained.

Some families will choose for the child to be at home for terminal care. This can be done with intense support from community nurses, the GP and hospital staff. Symptom relief is of paramount importance. The family should have contact numbers for any time of the day so that they feel well supported.

When the child dies, the family should be able to rely on the same team for support. They may need help with funeral arrangements. Continued bereavement care should be offered as the family will otherwise feel very isolated after the death of the child.

Medical aspects of splenectomy

Q. What are the clinical indications for splenectomy and what are the postoperative complications?

Indications for splenectomy can be divided into surgical and haematological causes.

1. *Surgical.* Traumatic rupture of the spleen is often cited as a surgical indication for removal as an emergency because of the risk of haemorrhage. In many cases this may be true, especially if the child is haemodynamically compromised, but limited surgery, i.e. splenorrhaphy, partial splenectomy or auto-transplantation may suffice. If the child is stable, continued monitoring with regular assessment of vital signs, serial haematocrits and spleen ultrasound/CT scanning may negate the need for surgery. Other surgical indications include spleno-renal shunting secondary to portal hypertension, splenic cysts and simply because the spleen has grown so large (e.g. Gaucher's disease)

2. *Haematological.* The list of potential indications is extensive; but include:
   — congenital haemolytic anaemias, e.g. hereditary spherocytosis, elliptocytosis
   — acquired immunohaematological conditions, e.g. autoimmunue haemolytic anaemia, ITP
   — Hodgkin's disease staging
   — sickle cell disease
   — hypersplenism, e.g. β-thalassaemia, Gaucher's

   a) *Sickle cell disease.* Acute splenic sequestration crisis is one of the leading causes of death in this condition. It occurs in homozygous 'sicklers' before the spleen is auto-splenectomised (aged 5 years maximum) and in older children with SC disease and S–B thalassaemia. Rapid enlargement of the spleen due to trapping of blood results in hypotension with cardiac decompensation. Treatment requires large volume blood transfusion. Some haematologists would consider one episode of acute splenic sequestration an indication for splenectomy once recovery has occurred; others two crises because of the risk of overwhelming sepsis in those without spleens.

   b) *Hodgkin's disease staging* (not undertaken in the UK). Ann Arbor staging III S for Hodgkin's disease requires splenectomy for histological analysis.

Currently, however, chemotherapy is given to virtually all children with Hodgkin's disease and therefore splenectomy is not indicated in the majority.

c) *Idiopathic thrombocytopaenic purpura.* 10–20% of ITP patients may have a chronic illness not responding to steroids, immunoglobulins or immunosuppressive agents (e.g. cyclophosphamide). In the past, splenectomy may have been performed if thrombocytopaenia persisted for longer than 6–12 months with a 65–87% chance of recovery of the platelet count. There is a move away from this as there is increasing evidence of spontaneous late recovery of the platelet count in ITP.

Postoperative complications

Overwhelming infection is the principle concern for patients post-splenectomy. They are particularly susceptible to *Streptococcus pneumoniae, Neiserria meningitidis, Haemophilus influenzae* and *Escherichia coli.* Risk is greater if there is an associated underlying disorder (e.g. β-thalassaemia, sickle cell disease) and also within the first 2–3 years after splenectomy. However, increased risk continues throughout life. Incidence of septicaemia is up to 4–5% and mortality is around 50%.

Ideally children should be vaccinated prior to splenectomy with polyvalent pneumococcal vaccine and subsequently every 5–10 years. Prophylactic penicillin (erythromycin if allergic) should be given daily for life. Immunisation with Hib vaccine would seem logical.

REFERENCES

McMillan M et al 1993 Long term management of patients after splenectomy. Br Med J 307: 1372–1373
Tait R C et al 1993 Late spontaneous recovery of chronic thrombocytopaenia. Arch Dis Child 68: 680–681

Treatment of thalassaemia

Q. What are the latest treatment guidelines for thalassaemia?

The β-thalassaemias are a group of haemoglobinopathies caused by deficient or absent β-globulin synthesis, occurring as a result of genetic mutations on chromosome 11. Principally in Mediterranean areas and Africa, carriers of thalassaemia genes have increased resistance to lethal *Plasmodium falciparum* malaria infection.

There are four clinical syndromes of increasing severity

— silent carrier
— thalassaemia trait
— thalassaemia intermedia
— thalassaemia major

The mainstay of treatment for *thalassaemic major* is *'hypertransfusion'* to maintain the haemoglobin above 10 g/dl. The reasons behind this are several fold:

1. Increased oxygen carrying capacity to prevent tissue hypoxia.
2. Switching off erythropoietin production in an attempt to reduce marrow expansion.
3. Promotion of normal growth and development by reducing the hypercatabolic state.
4. Reduction in gastrointestinal absorption of iron.

Some centres suggest 'super-transfusion', maintaining haemoglobin at 14 g/dl, This is a minority opinion, as it is known to increase the rate of iron loading. The frequency of blood transfusions can be reduced by transfusing neocytes, but these require increased blood donation from the general public (3 bags of packed cells = 1 bag of neocytes).

Complications of repeated blood transfusions exist:

1. Iron overloading.
2. Allergic reactions/anaphylaxis to transfusions.
3. Alloimmunisation producing haemolysis — detailed phenotyping of blood minimises this risk.
4. Viral infection transfer — hepatitis B, hepatitis C, HIV. Hepatitis B immunisation prior to starting transfusion is justified.

Iron overloading is the main indicator of prognosis. Without *chelation therapy*, cardiac haemosiderosis would prevent β-thalassaemia major sufferers reaching adulthood. No oral chelation therapies are available except on a research basis. In the UK, desferrioxamine is given subcutaneously. Because a pump is required to infuse the desferrioxamine, it is usually carried out at night when the child is asleep. In transfusion-dependant patients, chelation therapy should start by the age of 5 and some would advocate from the age of 3 years.

There are drawbacks to desferrioxamine infusions besides being very time consuming:

1. Local reactions — erythema, inflammation. Treatment by addition of hydrocortisone to the drug solution.
2. Neurosensory toxicity — includes high-frequency hearing loss and ocular toxicity. Formal audiometry and ophthalmological examination 6 monthly is recommended.

As well as regular blood transfusions and chelation therapy, ascorbic acid and folic acid should be prescribed. *Ascorbic acid* increases the amount of iron excretion in response to desferrioxamine and *folic acid* is given because of decreased absorption and increased requirement from the expanded bone marrow. Vitamin E supplementation may reduce the degree of haemolysis.

Cure for β-thalassaemia is possible by *bone marrow transplantation* (BMT), first described in 1982. If an HLA-matched donor can be found (1 in 4 chance of an identical sibling donor), studies from Italy show an 80% survival rate and 75% cure. Possibilities for the future besides BMT include gene therapies. Retroviral vectors may in the future be able genetically to transform the mutant bone marrow stem cells.

Splenectomy often becomes a necessity for β-thalassaemic major sufferer as a result of:

1. Hypersplenism.
2. Abdominal pain from the physical size of the spleen.
3. Increased requirement for blood transfusions.

The child should be vaccinated against pneumococcus prior to surgery and should remain on penicillin prophylaxis postoperatively ?for life.

Sickle cell disease

Q. A distressed 3-year-old girl of African origin is brought to casualty by her parents. She had been well until that afternoon when she suddenly cried out in pain and had been inconsolable since. On examination, she has a tender abdomen and splenomegaly. What would your management be now and in the future?

It is important to rule out the common causes of abdominal pain. I would want to be sure there was no history of abdominal trauma which might cause a *ruptured spleen*, with tender splenomegaly and pain. *Acute appendicitis*, *renal tract infection* or *mesenteric adenitis* might cause the pain, but a coincidental finding of splenomegaly would be unlikely. I would ask about a history of *sickle cell anaemia*, both in the child and other family members. A sequestration crisis in sickle cell anaemia may cause splenomegaly, but the spleen is often impalpable in a child of this age with sickle cell disease. Abdominal pain in a child with sickle cell disease is more often due to infarction or acute crisis than sequestration. It is important to ask about recent travel abroad, since the splenomegaly may easily be caused by malaria or kalaazar. I would also consider *glandular fever*, caused by Epstein Barr virus, in my differential diagnosis, although it would be an unusual presentation in this age group and with such acute pain.

Any of these illnesses may cause rapidly progressive hypotension and it is essential to gain venous access soon after admission. Blood pressure and pulse should be measured immediately and at frequent intervals. At the same time, I would take a full blood count and blood cultures and send a sample for urgent crossmatching. If I suspect sickle cell anaemia, I would send blood for haemoglobin electrophoresis. This should be done before any blood products are given. An urgent abdominal ultrasound should be performed to exclude splenic rupture. I would request the opinion of a paediatric surgeon to assist with diagnosis.

In both splenic rupture and sickle cell anaemia, the haemoglobin will have dropped and may be as low as 3 g/dl. Urgent blood transfusion is required. If the child shows signs of cardiovascular shock, such as agitation, extreme pallor, cool peripheries and hypotension, I would give a starting dose of 20 ml/kg of colloid, ideally plasma, while waiting for the blood. The child must be kept warm and I would also give oxygen. An acute crisis in sickle cell anaemia may be due to splenic sequestration in this age group. It is often secondary to infection, frequently by pneumococcus, so I would start intravenous antibiotics. Mortality in this condition is high and it is essential to maintain high fluid input to prevent shock.

Once stabilised, the child should be transferred to intensive care.

Splenectomy should be considered in splenic rupture or if the splenomegaly remains in sickle cell anaemia.

If sickle cell anaemia is confirmed, I would also suggest testing the parents and siblings. The child should be started on oral penicillin, even if she does not have a splenectomy, as there is a high incidence of overwhelming septicaemia due to pneumococcal infection. I would also give the pneumocooccal vaccine, since compliance with daily antibiotics is poor. This is not protective against all pneumococcal serotypes, but does afford some protection.

Education of the family is important. An affected child needs to be kept well hydrated during fever and in hot weather, and warm in cold weather, in an attempt to prevent further crises. The child should be given a card to carry saying that she has sickle cell disease in case she becomes unwell.

Screening, both antenatally and in the newborn period, is available. The risk of another affected child should be explained to both parents by a genetic counsellor.

Petechial rash

Q. What are the causes of a purpuric rash in a child and how would you investigate this

The causes of purpura may be considered as

1. Abnormalities of platelets.
2. Abnormalities of vascular endothelium.
3. Abnormalities of clotting factors.

1. *Abnormalities of platelets* may be due to:

   a) Reduced production:
      — bone marrow failure including leukaemia, aplastic anaemias and as a drug reaction
      — isolated megakaryocyte failure, e.g. following viral infection
   b) Increased destruction:
      — immunological, e.g. idiopathic thrombocytopaenic purpura
      — infection, e.g. rubella, cytomegalovirus
      — consumption such as with disseminated intravascular coagulation or haemolytic uraemic syndrome, and with giant haemangiomas, i.e. Kasabach-Merritt syndrome
      — hypersplenism, e.g.thalassaemia and portal hypertension
   c) Abnormal platelet function:
      — drugs, e.g. aspirin
      — metabolic disorders such as in renal failure
      — inherited disorders, e.g. Von Willebrand's disease and Bernard-Soulier syndrome (abnormally large platelets). Ehlers-Danlos syndrome is also associated with abnormal platelet function

2. *Abnormalities of the vascular endothelium* may be due to:

   a) Infection — either bacterial, e.g. meningococcus or subacute bacterial endocarditis or viral, e.g. cytomegalovirus
   b) Henoch-Schönlein purpura
   c) Connective tissue disorders — rarely caused by systemic lupus erythematosus

3. *Abnormalities of clotting factors* may be either:

   a) Acquired — disseminated intravascular coagulation, malabsorption and liver disease
   b) Inherited — haemophilia A (factor VIII), haemophilia B (factor IX), Von

Willebrand's disease (factor VIII, VW factor and platelet dysfunction)

My investigations would be determined by the clinical picture. I would check a full blood count and film in all cases. The distribution of the purpuric rash is important and a rash confined mainly to the extensor surfaces of the lower limbs in a well child would suggest *Henoch-Schönlein purpura*. In this common disorder, I would monitor the blood pressure and check the urine for blood and protein.

In an unwell child, I would consider the diagnosis of *meningococcaemia* and immediately check blood cultures and start penicillin if this seemed likely. *Septicaemia* may cause disseminated intravascular coagulation and I would check a clotting screen, including fibrinogen degradation products. Pallor and a recent diarrhoeal illness may suggest *haemolytic uraemic syndrome* and I would check renal function.

If the diagnosis is not clinically obvious, further investigations will depend on the full blood count and film. If the platelet count is reduced, I would check for viral and bacterial infection. If pancytopaenia is present, I would arrange bone marrow aspiration. In idiopathic thrombocytopaenic purpura, the platelet count is usually very low and the history of bruising is short. If there is doubt about the diagnosis or the recovery is atypical, I would consider bone marrow aspiration.

If the platelet count is normal, I would check a clotting screen. Ideally, I would check bleeding time, but this is technically difficult to do. It is prolonged in thrombocytopaenia and with platelet dysfunction, e.g. Von Willebrand's disease. The prothrombin time (PT), which tests the clotting factors used in the extrinsic pathway, is prolonged in vitamin K deficiency, e.g. liver disease and malabsorption. The partial thromboplastin time (PTT), which tests the clotting factors involved in the intrinsic pathway, is increased in the haemophilias and Von Willebrand's disease. The thrombin time (TT) reflects the final common pathway in haemostasis and is prolonged in fibrinogen deficiency. Therefore in disseminated intravascular coagulation, the PT, PTT and TT will be greatly increased. If there is a family history of bleeding disorders or the clotting screen is suggestive of haemophilia, it is possible to measure the clotting factors individually.

Tip

■ The list of causes of purpura is not complete, but is intended to organise your thought processes! Remember that the cases you have seen are likely to be the most common and you should mention these first.

Swollen knee

Q. How would you investigate a child with a swollen knee?

I would first like to exclude *septic arthritis* as a cause, since this is easily treatable and severely destructive if allowed to progress. The child would be febrile and the joint swollen, hot to the touch and very tender. I would check the white cell count and ESR and take blood for culture. Ultrasound of the joint may confirm that an effusion is present. Joint aspiration should be undertaken to identify the organism, which is typically *Staphylococcus aureus*, coliforms, *Haemophilus influenzae* (less common now) or salmonellae (in sickle cell disease).

It is important to exclude *trauma* in the differential diagnosis, since this is the most common cause of a painful, swollen joint in childhood. A history of strenuous exercise may be the only 'trauma' elicited. Examination of the knee will reveal ligament injuries. Less commonly, X-ray will reveal bony injury, X-ray will also be helpful in the diagnosis of Osgood-Schlatter's disease, which is one of the osteochondroses and may present with localised swelling over the tibial tubercle.

Henoch-Schönlein purpura is a systemic vasculitis which is characterised by a purpuric rash predominantly on the lower limbs. Joint involvement is transient and may cause tenderness and sometimes swelling. I would check a full blood count and film, aiming to exclude leukaemia, which may present with arthralgia, though rarely swelling. The anti-streptolysin titre is positive in a third of cases, but this probably compares with the unaffected population at a similar age.

Reactive arthritis is a common cause of arthritis and occurs after viral infections, particularly rubella, mumps and glandular fever. However, it usually causes a polyarthritis. Viral titres can be taken; repeat samples will be required in the convalescent period.

Juvenile chronic arthritis (JCA) may present with single joint involvement, when it is known as pauciarticular-onset JCA. Rheumatoid factor is almost always negative. There are broadly two groups of children who present with pauciarticular JCA: mainly young girls who also develop iridocyclitis and often have antinuclear antibodies and mainly boys of about 9 years of age who are negative for antinuclear antibodies, but are positive for HLA B27. The latter may go on to develop ankylosing spondylitis in later life.

Autoantibody screening may also reveal antibodies to double stranded DNA, which is suggestive of *systemic lupus erythematosus*. There may also be a non-specific rash and renal involvement. I would find complement levels helpful in making the diagnosis since C3 and C4 may be low due to increased consumption. *Dermatomyositis* is another connective tissue disorder which may present with a swollen knee, but this is usually of insidious onset and occurs late in the disease. In this case the swelling is due to calcinosis and can be seen on X-ray. The creatine kinase may be high. Muscle biopsy confirms the diagnosis and shows degeneration of muscle fibres.

The arthritis of *acute rheumatic fever* usually affects the large joints and moves from joint to joint. The joint affected is usually very tender, swollen and red. The arthritis may be associated with subcutaneous nodules, erythema marginatum and carditis. Diagnosis is based mainly on clinical criteria, but is supported by a raised ESR, leucocytosis, positive throat culture for Group A streptococcus and a raised anti-streptolysin titre.

Children with *inflammatory bowel disease* may have large joint arthritis. The arthritis usually develops after the bowel symptoms, but is occasionally the presenting feature. The ESR will be raised. I would investigate the bowel disease where appropriate, as treatment of the primary condition usually improves the joint symptoms.

Psoriatic arthritis rarely presents in childhood and usually affects the small joints. Occasionally it causes a pauciarticular arthritis. HLA B27 may be positive in these cases.

Lyme disease causes a pauciarticular arthritis. It is typically associated with a prodromal febrile illness and characteristic rash, erythema chronicum migrans. It may be possible to elicit a history of a tick bite. If the history is suggestive, I would request antibody titre to borrelia burgdorferei.

Osteosarcoma may present with swelling of the knee, since the most commonly affected sites are the distal femur and the proximal tibia. The swelling is not usually painful, but may only have been noted following trauma. I would arrange an X-ray, which would show destruction of the usual bone pattern. Further investigation might include CT scan, technetium bone scan and bone biopsy.

Children with chronic illnesses may present with joint swelling, e.g. a haemophiliac may have joint swelling secondary to a bleed; a child with sickle cell disease may have joint swelling due to a painful crisis or salmonella infection. Further investigation of the joint may not be required. A child with cystic fibrosis may develop hypertrophic pulmonary osteoarthropathy, which can be diagnosed by demonstrating periosteal changes on X-ray or isotope bone scan.

Management of juvenile chronic arthritis

Q. How would you manage a child with juvenile chronic arthritis as an outpatient?

The child with juvenile chronic arthritis (JCA) needs regular assessment. I would record the number of joints affected, muscle wasting and the range of movement possible. Contractures may also be present. As with all chronic illnesses, general physical examination is important. This should include measurement of height and weight. I would examine the child for evidence of failure to thrive, skin rashes (including psoriasis), nail pitting, vasculitis and fever. Slit-lamp examination for chronic anterior uveitis should be performed on at least one occasion. I would check the urine for protein, since amyloidosis can occur rarely, and blood, which may be due to nephritis secondary to drug treatment.

I would take the opportunity to remind the patient and parents of the importance of daily exercise and physiotherapy in order to prevent disability at each clinic visit.

Treatment can be divided into:

1. Physical therapy
2. Drug therapy

The *physiotherapist* should be involved in the assessment and treatment of a child with arthritis from an early stage. The aims are:

— to maintain and improve the range of joint movement, thereby preventing deformity
— to increase joint stability
— to increase muscle bulk

Good motivation will be required from the child and family, since it is essential to follow an arduous *exercise programme*. For this reason, it is important to set realistic, and therefore achievable, goals and to set a schedule which fits into normal family life. It is important to maintain good general fitness. Swimming is a valuable form of exercise, since it offers the chance to exercise the joints with less resistance from gravity, while being fun. Passive exercise is employed when the joints are acutely inflamed.

Splints may be useful to the child with chronic arthritis. Resting splints will relieve pain in inflamed joints while maintaining good joint position. Functional splints may be useful for some children, e.g. a wrist splint in the child who has discomfort while writing. Corrective splints are infrequently required in chronic arthropathy in children.

Non-steroidal anti-inflammatory drugs (NSAIDs) are the mainstay of drug treatment in juvenile arthritis. They are indicated in those with active synovial inflammation. The exact mode of action is unclear, but they are thought to work by inhibition of prostagladin synthesis. The dose used is generally higher per kilogram than that used in adults. There are numerous different NSAIDs. I tend to use just a few, so that I am familiar with the side-effects. However, some children will respond to one better than another. I treat the child with generous doses for a couple of months before changing to another type if the response is poor. Medication should be continued for 6 months after the inflammation has settled. Side-effects include rash, abdominal pain (including gastric ulceration), mood alterations and interstitial nephritis.

If a single joint is badly affected, disease remission may be relieved by intra-articular injection of *corticosteroids*, such as triamcinolone. This can be done under general anaesthetic. It may cause skin atrophy.

Disease-modifying drugs are rarely required in childhood, since the response to NSAIDs is usually so good and seem to be less effective in children than in adults. Methotrexate is the most useful and is given orally in low doses with response in 70% of patients. The patient should be monitored for liver and renal dysfunction, as well as bone marrow depression. There does not seem to be an increased risk of future neoplasia or infertility. Penicillamine and hydroxychloroquine do not seem to have any beneficial effect in juvenile arthritis. Intramuscular gold has occasionally been used in children, but it has not been thoroughly tested. Sulphasalazine is under investigation as a useful second-line drug in children, but its use may be limited by side-effects.

Finally, oral corticosteroids have a role in the treatment of systemic arthritis when anaemia or pericarditis are present. They should be used with caution due to the severity of the side-effects.

Clinical pharmacology and therapeutics

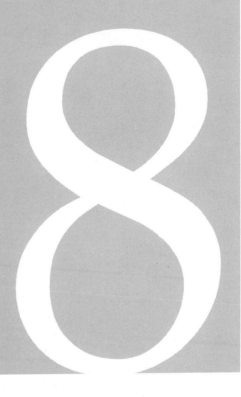

8

Drug interactions

Q1. What can you tell me about drug interactions?

A drug interactions is defined as an alteration in the effect of one drug by another which may be deleterious or beneficial. The possibility of drug interaction should be considered when any new drug is added to an existing treatment regimen and, clearly, the greater the number of drugs the child is receiving, the greater the potential for serious drug interactions. Drug interactions are particularly important in the very young child, in severe illness or in organ failure, such as renal, hepatic or cardiac, or when introducing drugs with a narrow therapeutic index. Adverse drug interactions may be divided into *pharmacokinetic* and *pharmacodynamic*. Pharmacokinetics refers to the body's handling of drugs, i.e. absorption, distribution, metabolism and excretion (what the body does to the drug). Pharmacodynamics refers to the biological effects of drugs, including their therapeutic effects (what the drug does to the body).

Q2. Tell me about some pharmacokinetic interactions.

Pharmacokinetic interactions are probably very common but. of clinical significance relatively infrequently in paediatric practice. The first site of possible interaction is intraluminal complexing in the unusual situation of a child on antacids where there may be interference with iron or prednisolone absorption. Again, in the unusual situation of a child on cyclosporin, erythromycin may almost double its absorption which may be related to inhibition of its partial metabolism in the gastric mucosal wall. A girl on the oral contraceptive pill will be at risk of pregnancy if she is given a course of broad-spectrum antibiotics (e.g. amoxycillin) which destroy gut bacteria. This is because enterohepatic recirculation, which increases plasma levels, is dependant on gut-floral deconjugation of pill hormones.

Various drugs such as corticosteroids, warfarin and oral contraceptives are metabolised by hepatic enzymes. *Enzyme inducers* such as anticonvulsants (phenytoin, carbamazepine and phenobarbitone) and rifampicin will attenuate their plasma levels, although this may take 2–3 weeks for maximal effect since it is dependant on increased protein synthesis.

Some drugs such as erythromycin, metronidazole, chloramphenicol, isoniazid and sodium valproate have *enzyme-inhibition* properties which may cause dangerous potentiation of other drugs such as warfarin, phenytoin, carbamazepine and theophylline. With both enzyme inducers and inhibitors, the opposite pharmacological effect should be anticipated if the drug is withdrawn after a period of administration.

Plasma–protein binding displacement will produce a transient rise in the plasma level of a drug but this will be accompanied by a compensatory rise in metabolism or excretion. The steady-state levels before and after addition of the displacing drug will therefore be similar. This mechanism applies to the potentiation of phenytoin by sodium valproate. Incidentally, this also applies to potentially dangerous displacement of bilirubin from plasma proteins in the neonate by drugs such as sulphonamides which may lead to kernicterus.

Interference with renal excretion is clinically significant if the drug is water-soluble, so that a large fraction is excreted unchanged. There may be dangerous potentiation of aminoglycoside toxicity (VIIIth nerve damage and nephrotoxicity) with cephalosporins or loop diuretics.

Q3. What do you know about pharmacodynamic interactions?

Pharmacodynamic mechanisms involve interactions between two drugs at sites of biological effects and may be usefully divided into synergistic and antagonistic.

Dangerous *synergistic* sedative effects can occur with any of the CNS-depressant drugs such as benzodiazepines, tricyclic antidepressants, antihistamines, phenothiazines (and ethanol).

Non-steroidal anti-inflammatory drugs reduce platelet adhesiveness and will therefore tend to potentiate the haemorrhagic tendency induced by warfarin (in addition, they may cause bleeding from mucosal damage in the gastrointestinal tract). Potassium supplementation increases the tendency to hyperkalaemia induced by angiotensin-converting enzyme inhibitors. Diuretic-induced hypokalaemia will increase the risk of arrhythmias caused by digoxin.

There are several examples of pharmacodynamic *antagonism* such as vitamin K and warfarin and β_2-agonists (e.g. salbutamol) and β_2- blockers. A less obvious but equally important effect is the antagonism of bactericidal antibiotics, such as penicillins or aminoglycosides, by bacteriostatic antibiotics, such as tetracyclines (e.g. in older adolescents on anti-acne therapy).

Q4. What do you understand by first-pass metabolism?

First-pass metabolism describes the metabolic breakdown of a drug en route between the gut and the systemic circulation (via the portal vein) during its first pass through the liver. An orally-administered drug which has a high first-pass metabolism will have low bioavailability.

Examples of drugs which show high first-pass metabolism are β_2-agonists (salbutamol and terbutaline), analgesics (aspirin, codeine and morphine), prochlorperazine, chlormethiazole, oral contraceptives and mebendazole. Enzyme-inducers increase hepatic blood flow and therefore further reduce the bioavailability of these drugs.

Tip

■ A difficult, rather technical question! The above should give you a broad structure which you can use to discuss other interactions you may have encountered. Once again, a logical approach is far more important than numerous examples.

Drugs in pregnancy

Q1. Tell me about the potential adverse effects of drugs on the fetus.

The taking of medication in pregnancy is a particularly sensitive subject which was highlighted by the worldwide reporting of thalidomide teratogenesis in the 1960s. Despite this, information on the risks of drugs in pregnancy is rather sparse and for ethical reasons has to be collected in a haphazard fashion, mostly by the 'yellow-card' system. Although a paediatrician will have no control over the administration of drugs in pregnancy, it is important that he/she has a working knowledge of the potential effects on the child and should accordingly be fully informed of exposure to such drugs by the obstetrician.

The only commonly used drugs which do *not* cross the placenta are heparin (because of its large molecular size) and curare (because of its polarity). The rest have access to the fetus and therefore the potential to affect growth and development. The harm that medications may cause to the unborn child may be classified into teratogenic and fetal effects.

Q2. Tell me about teratogenicity.

Teratogenicity refers to the potential of a drug to interfere with the process of *organogenesis* in the fetus. This occurs during the embryonic period and lasts from the 4th to the 10th week of gestation (which is the 2nd to the 8th week of conception). Various drugs are definitely known to be teratogenic from either animal study data or from reported human cases. Many more are not known to be definitely safe and therefore should be generally avoided in pregnancy until a sufficient pool of safety data has been accumulated from sporadic exposure. This applies to most new drugs.

Thalidomide was used as a hypnotic/sedative and is the best known of all human teratogens. Administration between 6 and 8 weeks gestation has resulted in phocomelia involving absence of limb long bones. It is still occasionally used in non-pregnant women as a anti-tuberculous drug.

Most currently used anticonvulsants have teratogenic properties. *Phenytoin* (a hydantoin) is well known for causing the fetal hydantoin syndrome which comprises craniofacial abnormalities, such as cleft lip and palate, hypertelorism and a broad nasal bridge hypoplasia of the distal phalanges and nails, growth impairment and mental retardation. Studies suggest that one-third of all babies born to mothers who were given phenytoin in early pregnancy had minor abnormalities such as cleft lip and 10% had major defects. Phenytoin teratogenicity appears to be at least partly genetically mediated since it 'runs true' in subsequent generations and may only affect one set of dizygotic twins.

Sodium valproate induces neural tube defects in 1–2% of pregnancies. In addition, it has occasionally been associated with abnormalities of the face and digits in the fetal valproate syndrome. Carbamazepine is generally considered to be the safest anticonvulsant in pregnancy and many epileptic women are switched to this therapy if they are planning to become pregnant. However, it may rarely be associated with a similar range of congenital abnormalities as phenytoin. Epilepsy is a difficult problem in pregnancy and, generally speaking, the risk to the fetus of maternal fits is greater than the teratogenic effects of anticonvulsants. In addition, there is some evidence that epilepsy itself is associated with fetal abnormalities.

The coumarin anticoagulant *warfarin* is a small molecule and readily crosses the placento-fetal barrier. If administered in the first trimester of pregnancy, it is associated with the so-called fetal warfarin syndrome which consists of nasal hypoplasia and epiphyseal stippling together with various other features such as hydrocephaly or microcephaly and growth and/or developmental delay. This occurs in about 15–20% of cases where there has been first-trimester exposure.

The *retinoids* such as isotretinoin are increasingly used systemically for severe acne and are also well-known teratogens. They are derivatives of vitamin A and are contraindicated in pregnancy though one occasionally sees cases where there has been exposure. They can cause severe congenital abnormalities including heart defects, cerebral and ocular defects, microtia, micrognathia and thymic agenesis. Approximately one-third of early exposures will result in significant abnormalities.

Lithium in early pregnancy is associated with a variety of cardiac defects (8% have severe disease), including the otherwise rare Epstein's anomaly which occurs in 3% of cases.

Various hormones have been reported as having teratogenic properties. The best known of these is *diethylstilboestrol* (DES) which is a synthetic oestrogen which can lead to vaginal clear-cell adenocarcinoma in the female offspring of women whose mothers were given the drug in pregnancy in late embryogenesis. *Tetracycline* is the only commonly used antibiotic definitely known to have teratogenic properties, causing yellow-brown discoloration of deciduous teeth and bones. It does not, however, increase the incidence of caries, nor does it cause impairment of bone growth. Many anti-neoplastic drugs have teratogenic properties though these drugs are generally only used if absolutely necessary. Examples are methotrexate (short stature and craniosynostosis), busulphan (growth retardation, cleft lip and ocular defects) and cyclophosphamide (growth retardation and cleft lip).

Q3. OK, I'll stop you there. Tell me about non-teratogenic damage.

Non-teratogenic effects or 'fetal effects' of drugs are related to damage to organs after they have been normally initiated and formed during the embryonic phase. Several drugs are associated with 'fetal effects' but may still be indicated if the benefits outweigh the potential risks.

In the second or third trimester, *warfarin* may result in fetal intracerebral haemorrhage, microcephaly and cataracts. Despite the potential adverse effects, warfarin is often used outside the embryonic phase and the immediate preterm period (when heparin is prefered) in pregnant women with significant thromboembolic risk. (Heparin is too large to cross the placenta but prolonged use is associated with a high incidence of maternal side-effects, notably osteoporosis and thrombocytopaenia.)

Sulphonamides in late gestation may compete with bilirubin for protein binding and cause neonatal hyperbilirubinaemia.

Trimethoprim is a weak folate antagonist, though convincing evidence of fetal damage has not been demonstrated.

Prolonged use of *aminoglycosides* in pregnancy may lead to fetal ototoxicity in approximately 2% of cases.

β-blockers may predispose to intrauterine growth retardation, fetal bradycardia and hypoglycaemia. *Angiotensin-converting-enzyme inhibitors* are associated with renal defects and anuria. *Thiazide diuretics* predispose to neonatal thrombocytopaenia.

Aspirin has been associated with haemorrhagic disorders and premature closure of the ductus if used in analgesic doses. *Opioid analgesics* if used in large doses around delivery, may cause neonatal respiratory depression which will reverse with naloxone.

Drugs and breastfeeding

Q. What do you know about maternal drug therapy and breastfeeding?

The vast majority of drugs are excreted in breast milk but in amounts that are too small to harm the baby. Milk/plasma concentration ratios vary from 0.3 to 1.0 depending on drug solubility, pH and dose interval. Most commonly used drugs in the puerperium can be safely administered to a mother who is breastfeeding and specifically penicillins, cephalosporins, Augmentin, most non-narcotic analgesics, insulin, methyldopa, commonly used anticonvulsants (such as sodium valproate, phenytoin and carbamazepine), frusemide, digoxin and β-blockers are all considered *safe*. Both heparin and warfarin appear to be safe but phenindione should be avoided because of the risk of neonatal haemorrhage.

Some drugs are, however, potentially harmful to the neonate and should either be *avoided* or *breastfeeding discontinued* if administration is deemed necessary. Examples are:

Cytotoxics	— cytotoxicity
Carbimazole	— suppression of neonatal thyroid
Amiodarone	— neonatal thyroid toxicity
Lithium	— hypotonia and cyanosis
Ergotamine	— neonatal ergotism
Barbiturates	— drowsiness
Benzodiazepines	— drowsiness
Chloramphenicol	— bone-marrow toxicity and 'grey syndrome'
Aspirin	— Reye syndrome and hypoprothrombinaemia
Indomethacin	— one reported case of neonatal convulsions
Laxatives	— neonatal diarrhoea
Prednisolone	— continuous therapy with >10 mg daily may affect the infant's adrenal gland

Tips

■ A problem which is poorly understood but one which you are likely to have encountered frequently during those numerous trips to the postnatal wards!

■ To illustrate your answer pick out some of the 'no go' drugs from the list of problem ones you have met yourself.

Adenosine

Q. What can you tell me about the drug adenosine?

Adenosine can be administered intravenously in paroxysmal *supraventricular tachycardia*. It acts by slowing conduction of the electrical impulse through the atrioventricular node. This action can interrupt re-entry circuits and thereby restore sinus rhythm in patients with paroxysmal supraventricular tachycardia, e.g. in the Wolff-Parkinson-White syndrome. In this case, once the circuit has been broken, the tachycardia should stop and sinus rhythm be re-established. It is useful in any supraventricular tachycardia since it slows down the ventricular rate, thus revealing the underlying atrial rhythm. However, it does not convert atrial flutter or fibrillation to sinus rhythm.

Adenosine is useful in an emergency, when supraventricular tachycardia is causing cardiovascular compromise. It is given intravenously by rapid bolus injection, while using a cardiac monitor. Although no controlled trials have been performed in children, it seems to be effective and safe in a dose of 0.25 mg/kg. If the first dose is not effective in reducing the ventricular rate, a second, then third dose can be given after a few minutes. The half-life of adenosine is very short — a matter of seconds — so a larger dose should be safe. Side-effects include facial flush, headaches and lightheadedness. As the tachycardia converts to sinus rhythm, ventricular ectopics, bradycardias and atrioventricular block may occur. Although unnerving, these are transient. Atropine is not effective if bradycardia occurs secondary to adenosine, but due to the short half-life, these should be fleeting.

In summary, adenosine is used intravenously with good effect in paroxysmal supraventricular tachycardias and is also helpful in the diagnosis of other rapid supraventricular tachycardias.

Tips

■ It is important to start off confidently. You may know very little about the drug itself, but try to think back quickly to when you have seen it used. What were the indications and how quickly did it work?

■ Divert onto the physiology of impulse conduction in the heart if you feel your knowledge is adequate.

■ Admit to little experience with adenosine by all means, but he prepared then to talk about your own method of treating paroxysmal SVT.

New anticonvulsants

Q. What can you tell me about new drugs used in the treatment of children with epilepsy?

Traditional anticonvulsants are successful in the treatment of at least 80% of epileptics. There was a long period with no development of new anticonvulsants but recent interest in modifying the neuronal hyperexcitability which causes epileptic discharge has lead to the manufacture of new drugs thought to act by altering the concentration of neurotransmitters within the brain. Trials of these drugs have been on patients with chronic intractable epilepsy who are already on a variety of anticonvulsants. This makes it difficult to assess the use of the new drugs as first-line agents and they are currently only licensed for use when other treatments have failed to control seizures.

Vigabatrin is the first drug specifically designed to alter neuronal excitability. It binds to GABA aminotransferase and prevents the breakdown of GABA, an inhibitory neurotransmitter. It has been shown to reduce seizure frequency by 50% in those with partial seizures, with or without generalisation. Although it has a short half-life and is cleared unchanged by the kidneys, it can be given once or twice daily since it is bound irreversibly to the enzyme. Side-effects include drowsiness, weight gain and behavioural problems. These may be reduced by slow introduction, but vigabatrin should be avoided in people with a history of mental illness, since it can cause a psychotic reaction. There has been some concern about the long-term safety of vigabatrin, as it has been shown to produce changes in the white matter of rats. The significance of these changes is unknown as they have not been demonstrated in humans. *field defied*

Gabapentin is a GABA-related amino acid and therefore acts as an inhibitory neurotransmitter. It has been shown to be useful in the control of generalised tonic-clonic convulsions.

Lamotrigine is thought to act by reducing the release of glutamate, which is an excitatory neurotransmitter. In this way it stabilises neuronal membranes. It has been used in partial seizures, especially if there is generalisation. It may also be useful in the most resistant epileptic syndromes, such as Lennox-Gastaut syndrome. It is metabolised in the liver before excretion, so sodium valproate will prevent its metabolism, while phenytoin will accelerate it. Side-effects include headache, ataxia and a rash, which may improve without withdrawal of the drug, but rarely develops into Stevens-Johnson syndrome. Lamotrigine is not yet licensed for use in children under 12 years of age.

Tips

■ You may know very little about the drugs mentioned. If possible, divert the examiners, e.g. the mention of Lennox-Gastaut syndrome may provoke an interrogation on its definition. As always, however, do not introduce something you know nothing about.

■ Enzyme induction/inhibition is a useful piece of pharmacology to know, especially if asked about anticonvulsants.

Adverse effects of carbamazepine

Q1. You've probably used carbamazepine on a number of occassions in childhood epileptic disorders. Tell me about its possible adverse effects.

Carbamazepine is a drug of choice for generalised tonic–clonic seizures and for simple and complex partial seizures with a wider therapeutic index. It generally has fewer adverse effects compared to phenytoin. (It is not used for absence seizures.)

Most of the more commonly encountered adverse effects are mild and either transient or reversible. It can occasionally, however, cause more serious reactions. I would group the possible adverse effects by system:

1. *Neurological.* Mild degrees of unsteadiness are dose-related and may be dose-limiting. Occasionally carbamazepine-induced exacerbation of seizures, particularly generalised absence seizures, can occur. Multiple tics and vocalisations are rarely seen 2–4 weeks after starting therapy and may occur within the therapeutic range. Extrapyramidal reactions such as dystonic movements and oculogyric crisis and impairment of peripheral nerve function have also been described.

2. *Dermatological.* A non-specific erythematous maculopapular eruption is relatively common and represents one of the milder hypersensitivities. More serious reactions are Stevens-Johnson syndrome, toxic epidermal necrolysis, exfoliative dermatitis and drug-induced systemic lupus erythematosus.

3. *Haematological.* Leukopaenia occurs in about 12% of children treated with carbamazepine and usually occurs within 3 months of commencement. The effect usually reverses even if therapy is continued and monitoring of the blood count is generally not indicated. However, regular FBCs are recommended in children with low or low/normal pre-treatment white cell counts. Rarely, more serious bone marrow depression with agranulocytosis or even pancytopaenia can occur. Other rare adverse effects include haemolytic anaemia, reticulocytosis (in the absence of bleeding or haemolysis) and thrombocytopaenia.

4. *Hepatic.* Granulomatous hepatitis presenting with pyrexia, sweats, abdominal pain and jaundice may occur but is reversible on discontinuing

treatment. Fatal hepatic failure in one girl has been described as has cholestatic jaundice.

5. *Cardiovascular.* Carbamazepine may occasionally exert inhibitory properties on the cardiac conducting system and therefore cause atrioventricular block and bradyarrhythmias.

6. *Metabolic.* Carbamazepine is a well known cause of drug-induced hyponatraemia due to inappropriate ADH secretion.

7. *Respiratory.* There are case reports of acute eosinophilic pulmonary hypersensitivity reactions.

For the above reasons, I would commence carbamazepine at a low dose and aim to increase the regimen over about 2 weeks. I would avoid using it in children with pre-existing hepatic, renal or cardiac disease and I would use it with caution in those with haematological disease.

Q2. Do you know anything about is toxicity in overdosage?

The main problems are related to cardiac arrhythmias and conduction defects, seizures and chorea-like movements, respiratory depression and coma.

The management is generally supportive with close electrolyte and cardiac monitoring, gastric emptying and treatment of seizures with diazepam and phenytoin. I would consult with a poisons unit and if severe, manage the child on an intensive care unit.

Tip

■ Anticonvulsants are one of the commonest drug groups to be tested on. It is also worth brushing-up on corticosteroids and other asthma therapy and analgesics.

Adverse effects of inhaled steroids in asthma

Q. **Recent articles on asthma have moved practice towards the greater use of inhaled steroids. What do you know about the adverse effects of these preparations?**

Inhaled steroids are of central importance in the management of chronic asthma by markedly reducing the frequency and severity of acute attacks. They have been used to treat children with asthma for over 20 years. The terrible morbidity and mortality associated with this very common disease is therefore significantly improved by their prophylactic effects. However, because of the obvious side-effects of long-term oral steroids, many doctors have understandable concerns about the possible risks of the inhaled route. In addition, many parents are deeply anxious about the mere mention of the word steroid and will often be very probing about how the daily use of these drugs might affect their child.

In general terms, the side-effect profile of inhaled steroids is excellent in relation to their benefits. I would first like to consider *local* side-effects, largely to dismiss them since even though they are often reported in adults, they are rarely seen in paediatric practice. Oral colonisation by *Candida albicans* occurs in up to 50% of children using inhaled steroids (compared to 29% of controls) and does not appear to be significantly affected by the type of device used or by the dose. Clinical candidiasis, however, occurs in only a tiny fraction of these (1 out of 129 asthmatics in one study). Similarly, sore throat and hoarseness seems to be a very infrequent complication of inhaled steroids in children and is unrelated to candida. The theoretical adverse effects which evoke the greatest anxiety therefore relate to the *chronic* systemic absorption of inhaled steroids which may occur and these are still being evaluated. I would like to consider each of these in turn.

Growth has been the main area of concern. Several factors, including the effects of asthma itself, the ages of children studied and specifically the interaction of asthma, asthma treatment and pubertal growth, the type of study, compliance and practicalities of growth measurement, combine to mean that studies are generally complicated and inconclusive. The most important confounding problem is that there is no doubt that poorly controlled asthma itself impairs growth, at least temporarily. It was noted as early as the 1940s that children with moderate to severe asthma fall away from their predicated height centiles as they approach puberty (Cohen et al 1940). However, it was subsequently discovered that asthma also leads to delayed maturation by widening the prepubertal growth nadir. This essentially results in a more prolonged growth period and it has been demonstrated that most asthmatic children do in fact attain their predicted adult height (Balfour-Lynn 1986). Evidence also shows that controlling asthma with inhaled steroids can improve growth velocity (Ninan & Russell 1992).

In the opposite camp, Littlewood et al (1988) concluded that inhaled steroids can produce growth impairment but in fact many of the children in their study were of an age when pubertal changes would be expected to be significantly influencing growth. A more recent study (Ninan & Russell 1992) avoided this problem by only including prepubertal children (boys up to their 11th birthday and girls up to their 10th birthday). They could demonstrate no adverse effect on growth by inhaled steroids (dose range 200–1600 μg). Their findings also suggested that when growth impairment occurs in an asthmatic child, it is more likely to reflect poor asthma control than the administration of inhaled steroids.

Studies utilising short-term analysis of lower-leg growth velocity using a knemometer demonstrated reductions of about 0.2 mm per week with 400 μg/day of inhaled beclomethasone dipropionate. However, it is difficult to extrapolate these findings over longer periods and the data from long-term longitudinal studies is generally very reassuring.

The evidence relating to inhaled steroids and growth are therefore now fairly extensive but as yet still not conclusive. If I were counselling concerned parents regarding this matter, I would explain this and stress the following. First there is no doubt that poorly controlled asthma has inhibitory effects on growth, at least in the short term. Secondly, the long-term data on inhaled steroids is generally reassuring; and thirdly proper prophylactic control of their child's asthma with inhaled steroids should mean fewer courses of oral steroids which have many more definite risks.

Another bone-related concern which has caused increasing concern is a theoretical predisposition to osteoporosis in adult life. Osteoporosis is defined as reduced bone mass (both mineralised bone and unmineralised osteoid) per unit bone volume. Both the lay and the medical press have recently fielded numerous articles relating to this disabling condition. The rate of diagnosis in adults has reached epidemic levels in the Western world and it is now regarded as one of the major causes of disability and death in older adults. For example, it has been shown that an older woman suffering a fractured neck of femur has less than a 50% chance of returning to an independent existence.

The total bone mass in the older adult (and therefore the risk of osteoporosis) is determined by the peak bone mass and the rate of bone loss during life. With growth in early childhood, bone mass gradually increases in a linear fashion until puberty when a surge in growth velocity occurs. This lasts for about 3 years and in girls begins around 11 years and in boys around 14 years. Peak bone mass is finally achieved 3 or 4 years after this period of rapid pubertal growth. The final level of peak bone mass is determined by a variety of factors, the most important being genetic but also by various environmental factors such as physical activity, nutrition and calcium intake.

We know that long-term oral steroids predispose to osteoporosis by causing a reduction in total bone mass; in effect they worsen the age-related predisposition to osteoporosis. We also know that at doses sufficient to produce systemic absorption, inhaled steroids cause short-term, dose-related reductions in long bone growth velocity. Proof of long-term bone loss is, however, lacking. In addition, there is a hypothesis that inhaled steroids may have a second damaging action in children around the pubertal period, namely by reducing the peak bone mass that a child finally achieves. However, this is still open to debate and clinical evidence for peak bone mass reduction with inhaled steroids alone is lacking. All in all, there is as yet no firm evidence for inhaled steroids producing a predictable predisposition to osteoporosis in adult life. There does however appear to be marked individual variation in susceptibility with case reports of significant impairment at low doses (Priftis et al 1991). It may be that an unidentifiable group of children are at particular risk of the bone-damaging effects of corticosteroids.

Another important concern is *adrenocortical suppression*. The hypothalamic-pituitary-adrenal axis can be assessed by testing physiological secretion of corticosteroids and the adrenal response to stimulation. There are various reports of impairment of these tests with doses of beclomethasone dipropionate of 400–1000 µg/day. However, perhaps the most important finding is that clinical adrenal insufficiency has not been reported in adults or children treated with inhaled steroids alone.

Posterior subcapsular cataracts are a specific and well-recognised complication of long-term oral corticosteroid therapy. However, a Canadian study found no association with inhaled steroid therapy in children, even at moderate to high doses (Simons et al 1993). Also reassuring is the lack of evidence of significant disturbance of glucose or lipid metabolism in children on inhaled steroids. The easy bruising noted in adults on even low inhaled doses does not appear to be a problem in children.

It has long been realised that oral steroids can produce *psychiatric* and *behavioural disturbance*. However, such effects with inhaled steroids in children appear to be rare and are confined to case reports in the literature. Connet & Lenney (1991) described acute hyperactivity and tantrums in four children receiving 800–1200 µg of inhaled daily doses of budesonide.

In recent years, there has been increasing debate about the choice of inhaled steroid preparation for paediatric therapy. There is evidence that one of the newer preparations, fluticasone propionate, is twice as potent in its topical anti-inflammatory activity compared to beclomethasone. In addition, fluticasone is completely removed by first-pass metabolism in the liver when swallowed (about 80–90% of any inhaled drug is swallowed). However, systemic effects might theoretically arise from the fraction absorbed from the respiratory tract. In addition, despite the impressive in vitro profile of fluticasone, there is as yet little clinical evidence to support its proposed advantages over the older preparations (Drug and Therapeutics Bulletin 1994)

These findings show that many of the documented adverse effects of inhaled steroids in children have been in short-term studies or involve intricate biophysical measurements. Extrapolation of these effects to the patient as a whole have rarely been demonstrated and it is a mark of the general safety of inhaled steroids that unwanted clinical effects have so rarely been reported. There also appears to be a large body of evidence demonstrating the safety of inhaled steroids and their profoundly beneficial effects on chronic asthma.

However, theoretical risks remain and it is prudent to ensure that lowest effective doses of inhaled steroids are advised. Generally speaking, aerosol systems are appropriate for the more severe cases of asthma requiring steroid prophylaxis and spacer devices improve local pulmonary delivery and also reduce both local and systemic side-effects. Mouth washing after inhalation may help to reduce the tiny risk of oral candidiasis and may also reduce systemic absorption. Finally, children on inhaled steroids should have their symptoms, therapy inhaler technique and growth regularly reviewed.

Tip

■ This is a good example of casually leaving out some 'succulent bait' in the form of a brief diversion into osteoporosis. This is a 'hot topic' and one which parents will probably already have been briefed upon by the lay press. If you have a solid grasp of this field, your viva gamesmanship would direct you to introduce this topic. Hopefully you will be rewarded by the examiner taking the bait, perhaps by . . ." aah, osteoporosis isn't something that you or I will see much of but since you've raised it . . . why do you think it's important? . . . what do you know about its epidemiology?"

REFERENCES

Balfour-Lynn L 1986 Growth and childhood asthma. Arch Dis Child 61: 1049–1055

Cohen M B et al 1940 Anthropometry in children. Progress in allergic children as shown by increments in height, weight and maturity. Am J Dis Child 60: 1058–1066

Cohen M B, Abram L E 1948 Growth pattern of allergic children. Allergy 19: 165–171

Connet G, Lenney W 1991 Inhaled budesonide and behavioural disturbances. Lancet 338: 634

Drug and Therapeutics Bulletin 1994 32: 25–27

Geddes D M 1992 Inhaled corticosteroids; benefits and risks. Thorax 47: 404–407

Kelly P J et al 1990 The interaction of genetic and environmental influences on peak bone density. Osteoporosis Int 1990 1: 55–60

Littlewood J M et al 1988. Growth retardation in asthmatic children treated with inhaled beclomethasone diproprionate. Lancet i: 115–116

Ninan T, Russell G 1992 Asthma, inhaled corticosteroid treatment and growth. Arch Dis Child 67: 703–705

Priftis K, Everard M L, Milner A D 1991 Unexpected side effects of inhaled steroids: a case report. Eur J Pediatr 150: 448–449

Simons F E R et al 1993 Absence of posterior subcapsular cataracts in young patients treated with inhaled glucocorticoids. Lancet 342: 776–778

Malaria

Q1. What advice on prophylaxis would you give a mother taking her baby and 3-year-old on holiday to a malaria endemic area?

With increasing foreign travel, this is a question we are being asked more and more frequently.

The single most important thing for the mother to be told is that the best way of avoiding malaria is to ensure that the children avoid mosquito bites. I would explain this is how malaria is transmitted. To avoid bites, children need to sleep under mosquito nets which have preferably been impregnated with repellant chemical, or ensure netting is in place on windows. Mosquitos bite at dawn and dusk, as well as through the night, so at these times children, and indeed adults, should wear long trousers and sleeves, with mosquito repellant spray on the ankles and wrists.

In addition, the children will need to take *anti-malarial tablets*. The recommended medication varies with location, and recommendations frequently change. For an up-to-date opinion, I would consult the latest British National Formulary, or one of the Travel Advice Centres, such as the London School of Tropical Medicine and Hygiene. A typical recommendation for Kenya would be once weekly chloroquine and daily proguanil. These would be appropriate for both the toddler and infant. Chloroquine can be given as a syrup. I would have to look up the doses. Chloroquine resistance is now wide-spread, so if they were going to a resistant area, mefloquine would be an alternative for the older child. It is not recommended for use in children under 15 kg, or if there is a history of convulsions, and should not be taken for more than 3 months.

I would stress the need to *start* prophylaxis one week *before travelling*, to take it without fail on holiday, and to *continue* for at least 4 weeks after returning. This, I would explain, is important because symptoms may not develop before a few weeks after a bite.

It is also very important to stress that the protection is not absolute. If the children develop a fever or flu-like symptoms on holiday, or even several weeks or months after returning, this may be due to malaria, and the mother should seek medical help so that a blood film can be examined.

Q2. How would you treat them if they returned with malaria?

This is a *medical emergency*. Patients with malaria can deteriorate very quickly, and if they are clinically unwell, I would enlist expert help as soon as possible. The treatment depends on which *Plasmodium* parasite is responsible. If there is any doubt, I would treat as falciparum malaria, the most dangerous type. If the children have developed malaria despite chloroquine prophylaxis, then it is probably a chloroquine-resistant strain and I would treat with quinine. If the children can tolerate oral treatment, I would give a 7-day course of quinine followed by Fansidar, a mixture of pyrimethamine and sulfadoxine. Mefloquine and halofantrine are alternatives to quinine which need not be followed by Fansidar.

If the children are vomiting, or have a reduced level of consiousness, I would treat with intravenous quinine and give intravenous fluid. I would monitor the children carefully for complications of falciparum malaria, in particular hypoglycaemia and cerebral malaria. This is a reduced level of consciousness associated with fitting. Prophylactic phenobarbitone is recommended by some to prevent convulsions.

Benign malaria due to *Plasmodium vivax* or *Plasmodium ovale* can be treated with chloroquine. This must be followed by primaquine to clear the liver of any residual parasites which might otherwise give a later relapse. Before giving primaquine I would check that a child is not G6PD deficient.

Tip

■ This is a specialist area. The Membership candidate would not be expected to know the exact prophylactic recommendation for every country in the tropics. However, the principles of prophylaxis and treatment should be known.

Neurology, psychiatry, community paediatrics and ethics

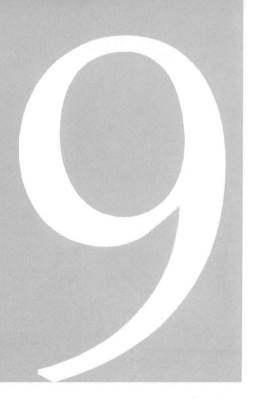

9

Cerebral palsy

Q1. What is your definition of cerebral palsy?

Cerebral palsy is a disorder of movement and posture due to non-progressive brain damage sustained by the immature brain. It is persistent but not static and the clinical features evolve throughout childhood. The motor function is not only delayed but also follows a course not seen in the normal child. Although the term cerebral palsy describes purely motor dysfunction, other parts of the brain may be affected by the same pathological process and associated features include epilepsy, mental retardation, visual and hearing impairment and specific learning problems.

Q2. Who do you think should be involved in the management of a child with cerebral palsy?

Cerebral palsy is a complex disorder and management requires the skills of many experts. At presentation, the child should be assessed by a multidisciplinary team in order to plan future management. This process of assessment will need to be repeated throughout childhood, since the pattern of motor deficit will constantly change.

A key member of the team will be a *physiotherapist*, who will work closely with the child and family after the diagnosis is made. Many physiotherapists specialise in paediatrics and have the most experience with physically handicapped children. It has been difficult to prove the effectiveness of early physiotherapy in cerebral palsy, due to a lack of suitable control subjects. However, it seems likely that early physiotherapy is of benefit to the child since it reduces the formation of contractures and harmful patterns of posture. The physiotherapist spends a lot of time with the child and therefore has the opportunity to teach the family how to handle the child in all aspects of daily living. The family will also learn the techniques used by the physiotherapist and will be able to continue exercises at home. There are many different methods of treatment, some of which are very intensive and time consuming. However, in practical terms, a method needs to be found which will allow the handicapped child to achieve a degree of independence and promote normal motor development, while fitting in to normal family life with minimal disruption to other children.

An *occupational therapist* will assess the child with respect to the activities of daily living. Changes to the family home may be required to make the child more independent, e.g. ramps for the wheelchair and cutlery designed for those with poor manipulative skills. Some children with cerebral palsy will have sensory deficits and the occupational therapist may be able to devise a sensory stimulation programme to accelerate the child's learning.

A *social worker* has an important role for the family. They may be able to suggest benefits which the parents are entitled to claim. They can be supportive in times of stress and may arrange short breaks for the child to give the family a rest. Sometimes it may be possible to arrange regular stays for the child with another family.

A *speech therapist* should be involved even before speech develops. They will assess the ability of the child to swallow and use the tongue and may be able to teach methods to inhibit reflexes which prevent normal feeding. Adequate nutrition may cause difficulty and failure of growth is a common problem. The *dietician* may be able to recommend a high calorie diet and if the child still fails to thrive, feeding may be achieved by nasogastric tube or gastrostomy.

Hearing and vision should be assessed by an *audiologist* and *ophthalmologist* respectively. Squints are common in cerebral palsy and correction may be beneficial.

An *orthopaedic surgeon* should work in close collaboration with the physiotherapist. Surgical intervention is rarely needed before the age of 5, but may then be useful in the correction of contractures and to improve posture.

Education of the child with cerebral palsy is important and a *teacher* will be involved in the assessment, in order to suggest what form of education the child will benefit from most. Many children with physical handicap also have learning difficulties and placement in a normal school may not be possible. However, it is essential that the child experiences social contact with his/her own age group. It is important to consider the practical difficulties, such as mobility, when choosing a school. The pre-school teacher will be able to help with stimulation of the child through toys and games.

Control of epilepsy with anticonvulsants and medication, such as baclofen, to reduce spasticity may be required. The *paediatrician* also needs to ensure that the skills of the various professionals are co-ordinated. Regular review of the child will highlight developing difficulties.

1. Physiotherapist
2. Occupational therapist
3. Speech therapist
4. dietician
5. Social worker
6. Audiologist
7. Ophthalmologist
8. orthopaedic surgeon
9. Paediatrician
10. School Teacher

Ataxia

Q. A 21-month-old boy has recently been ataxic. How would you proceed?

I would start with an accurate history. In acute onset ataxia, especially if fever is present, I would consider infection. Middle ear infection may cause a sensation of dizziness and corresponding ataxia. Persistent infection may spread to form a *cerebellar abcess*. Recent chickenpox infection might suggest *varicella encephalitis*.

It is important to consider *intoxication*, e.g. a child who has found the sherry or phenytoin bottle. Although unusual at this age, migraine may cause ataxia in young children and a family history of migraine should be sought.

If the onset of ataxia has been more prolonged, symptoms of raised intracranial pressure might suggest a structural problem and must be investigated urgently. My immediate priority would be to exclude a *posterior fossa tumour* which may be a medulloblastoma or astrocytoma. *Hydrocephalus* may be caused by a space-occupying lesion or aqueduct stenosis.

A much rarer cause of ataxia can also be suggested by the history; diarrhoea and malabsorption are symptoms of abetalipoproteinaemia, which is important as a potentially reversible cause of ataxia if a low-fat diet is instituted.

On examination I would search for cerebellar signs apart from ataxia, such as hypotonia, nystagmus, dysarthria and intention tremor. Proximal myopathy, e.g. in Duchenne muscular dystrophy, can give the impression of unsteadiness and therefore present as an ataxic gait. Muscle bulk and power should therefore be examined. Focal neurological signs may be indicative of the site of a tumour or infection and I would examine the eyes for telangectasia, although ataxia telangectasia usually presents at a later age.

Investigation will obviously be guided by the history. A white cell count may indicate infection. I would collect urine and blood samples for toxicology. In this age group I would proceed rapidly to cranial imaging, focusing particular attention on the posterior fossa. A MRI scan would be most useful if available. The scan should exclude hydrocephalus, arteriovenous malformation, cerebellar hypoplasia and tumours. It will also show loss of white matter suggestive of metachromatic leucodystrophy.

If no diagnosis is obvious, further investigations might include:

— Cholesterol and triglycerides (abetalipoproteinaemia)
— Immunoglobulins (ataxia telangectasia)
— Ammonia (urea cycle disorders)
— Urinary catecholamines (dancing eye syndrome and neuroblastoma)

Finally, I would repeat the head scan if no diagnosis is found, since the posterior fossa is notoriously difficult to visualise and the absence of a space-occupying lesion must be confirmed.

Hemiplegia

Q. What would you do with a 10-year-old child with sudden onset of left-sided weakness?

Prior to undertaking investigations, I would establish whether there had been any precipitating factors, e.g. trauma or convulsions. I would enquire about any family history of migraine, polycystic disease of the kidneys or hypertension. On examination, I would elicit the neurological signs and extent of weakness, in order to establish the anatomical site of the pathology. Examination of the fundi might reveal papilloedema suggestive of raised intracranial pressure. I would check the blood pressure and temperature. I would listen to the heart, as a septal defect might account for paradoxical emboli. I would look for cavernous haemangiomas superficially and also note capillary haemangiomas, particularly of the upper trigeminal region.

Causes of acute hemiplegia include:

1. *Trauma*. Head injury is the commonest cause of hemiplegia in children and may be due to subdural or extradural clot. Cerebral contusion or a contracoup injury also cause weakness. A rapidly deteriorating child with hemiplegia may have tentorial coning. Non-accidental injury should always be considered in an infant with hemiplegia.

2. *Vascular malformations*. Arteriovenous malformations are the commonest vascular lesions which present with hemiplegia in children. They are usually unilateral and 50% are in the parietal area. There is a high risk of haemorrhage. Cavernous haemangiomas are mostly supratentorial and in the territory of the middle cerebral artery. They may cause intracerebral or subarachnoid haemorrhage. The capillary haemangiomas associated with Sturge-Weber syndrome usually present with epilepsy and rarely bleed. Cerebral aneurysms may be familial, or associated with coarctation of the aorta, Ehlers-Danlos syndrome and polycystic disease of the kidneys. Many are idiopathic. They present as subarachnoid bleeds, which may in turn cause secondary cerebral infarction.

3. *Vascular occlusions*. Thrombosis may be secondary to hypercoagulable states. Polycythaemia in the child is usually due to cyanosis, e.g. in the child with congenital heart disease or chronic lung disease. Hyperviscosity may also be due to severe dehydration. Children with poorly controlled diabetes mellitus with ketoacidosis and hyperlipidaemia may also develop thrombosis. In the extremely unwell child with septicaemia or haemolytic uraemic syndrome, vascular occlusion may occur secondary to disseminated intravascular coagulopathy. A child with sickle cell disease may present with hemiplegia

caused by vascular occlusion. Rarely, abnormalities of the plasma proteins, S and C, cause a hypercoagulable state and present with stroke. Arteritis due to the connective tissue disorders, especially systemic lupus erythematosus, may cause any neurological lesion, including hemiparesis.

Emboli of blood clots, fat, air or vegetations from cardiac lesions may cause vascular occlusion and stroke. The source of the emboli is usually the heart or neck vessels, but in congenital heart disease with septal defects the emboli may derive from pelvic vessels.

4. *Infection.* Viral encephalitis rarely causes hemiplegia, the exception being herpes simplex encephalitis, which typically causes temporal lobe signs but may be focal and cause an acute hemiplegia in older children. Early diagnosis is important since it is a treatable cause. Toxoplasmosis should be considered, particularly if there is a risk of immunosuppression in the child. Bacterial meningitis can cause hemiplegia by thrombosis of the cortical blood vessels. Post-infectious encephalitis due to mumps, measles and varicella may present acutely with hemiplegia. A cerebral abscess from middle ear infection should also be considered.

5. *Ischaemia.* Status epilepticus, cardiac arrest, near drowning and acute hypotension, e.g. due to blood loss or septicaemia, may all cause hemiplegia, but would usually be associated with more global deficits. Temporary hemiplegia may occur postictally in epilepsy (Todd's paresis).

6. *Neoplasia.* Haemorrhage into a tumour, e.g. a glioma, may cause sudden weakness. Meningeal leukaemia is less common with modern treatment protocols but haemorrhage may occur due to thrombocytopaenia.

7. *Migraine.* Sudden onset of unilateral weakness, with or without sensory symptoms, may be the presenting feature of migraine. It may be associated with dysarthria or aphasia. The prognosis is usually good with complete recovery within hours or days. There may be a family history and the attacks may be recurrent but tend to stop in adult life.

My investigation of this child would depend on the history given, but I would like to arrange an urgent cranial CT scan in most cases. The results of the scan would guide me with respect to further investigation. Initial blood tests might include a full blood count with packed cell volume measurement, clotting studies, blood culture and virology titres. EEG would be helpful in the diagnosis of encephalopathic disorders. An echocardiogram would be indicated in a child with a heart murmur. Cerebral angiography is invasive but may be necessary to identify bleeding sites and the extent of arteriovenous malformations prior to surgery. MRI angiography is a less invasive method of diagnosing arterial or venous occlusion. Further blood tests to look for causes of vasculitis or hypercoagulable states may be necessary.

Lead poisoning

Q. What can you tell me about lead poisoning in children?

The Centers for Disease Control and Prevention (CDC) in October 1991 issued a statement on lead, suggesting the need for universal screening for blood lead determinations and describing lead as the number one environmental health issue for American children. Lead is a toxic metal that has no function in humans. Up until the mid-18th century, atmospheric lead was minimal, but since then there has been a rapid increase, especially since the 1930s when lead was added to petrol as an anti-knock agent. There are several sources of lead:

1. Air: ~55 000 tons a year are released into the atmosphere by motor vehicles in the US. Since the introduction of lead-free petrol, this figure has dropped
2. Food and water: especially from canned foods (lead solder)
3. Paint: pre-war (WWII) paint contained up to 40% lead by dry weight. Peeling and flaking paint is easily transferred from walls to children's mouths!
4. Miscellaneous: Farouk — Saudi Arabian remedy to enhance teeth eruption; Al Kohol/surma — cosmetic paints; Bint at Zahab — treatment of colic in Saudi Arabia; old battery casings; lead painted toys, etc.

The effects of lead are principally on the mitochondria, causing:

— inactivation of enzymes
— interference with haem synthesis
— interference with vitamin D metabolism
— protoporphyrin accumulation in glial cells and demyelination
— inhibition of synthesis of cytochrome P-450

Symptoms and signs of lead poisoning are non-specific and, although a rare cause, must be thought of in children with anaemia, fits, behavioural and learning difficulties, abdominal pain and vomiting. A child admitted in acute encephalopathy with punctate basophilia and anaemia, amino aciduria and Fanconi's syndrome and speckling of his/her gut on plain abdominal X-ray is a little easier to diagnose correctly.

The American Academy of Pediatrics recommends blood lead testing as part of routine health surveillance in all 10–14 month olds and again at 2 years of age. There are no such recommendations in the UK as the financial implications must be awesome, never mind the administration of such a policy. Whether or not there is a fine balance between screening all children and simply screening those with the non-specific signs and symptoms mentioned above is debatable. If like many aspects of medicine in Britain we lag behind the US by several years, then lead poisoning in children will become the next 'fad' (after cholesterol and triglyceride levels!)

REFERENCE

Schonfield D J 1993 New developments in paediatric lead poisoning Curr Opin Ped 5: 537–544

Chronic fatigue syndrome

Q1. Tell me your thoughts on chronic fatigue syndrome in children?

Prolonged fatigue, usually occurring after a viral infection, has variously been named myalgic encephalomyelitis (ME), postviral fatigue syndrome and, more recently, chronic fatigue syndrome. It has caused controversy in the medical literature for over 50 years. It has also been termed The Royal Free Disease after one of the early documented reports. In 1955, a doctor and a ward sister at that hospital complained of a strange fatigue-producing illness that ultimately affected so many staff that the hospital had to be closed temporarily. The condition was originally described in adults but an increasing number of children have been labelled with the diagnosis in recent years.

The diagnosis is a purely clinical one. The typical picture is *fatigue*, which may be progressive, occurring with defined onset, usually following a viral infection such as an influenzal or coryzal illness. I would define fatigue as a sensation of tiredness or weariness occurring at rest. These patients may also report undue fatiguability with physical or mental exertion. Various associated symptoms have been described, such as headache, myalgia, difficulty concentrating, somnolescence, dizziness, nausea and sore throat. Most patients also have emotional symptoms with depression, tearfulness, irritability and anxiety.

Another important feature is the remarkable absence of constant or reproducible manifestations of physical abnormality, either on thorough general and neurological clinical examination or extensive investigation. Over the years, minor abnormalities found in complex investigations have been reported in adults (muscle biopsies, enzyme studies and MRI scans). Parents or patients are often quick to latch onto these and may even come to clinic armed with original articles in order to lend 'organic validity' to these symptoms. However, the consensus medical view is that no consistent abnormality has been found on investigating these patients and there is no convincing evidence for an organic causation.

The increasing recognition of the illness in paediatrics has led to considerable concern because of the potentially devastating specific effects in children, such as absence from school, restricted physical, psychological and social development and the development of long-term psychological illness.

Margaret Vereker has attempted to provide a clinical description and plan of management of chronic fatigue syndrome in paediatrics in her study of 10 affected children. Criteria used in her study were a definable onset such as following a viral infection, generalised fatigue, fatiguability, associated symptoms such as headache, interference with general functioning and lack of demonstrable organic illness after appropriate assessment by a paediatrician or another consultant. The criteria of duration in adult studies is usually 6 months but this was felt to be inappropriately long for paediatric practice and 6 weeks was used. Her management plan involved a joint paediatric–psychiatric approach with general and community paediatricians, child psychiatrists and psychologists.

Some of the children were found to have such severe restriction of motor function as to produce difficulty in walking or even paralysis. However, it was noted by both medical and nursing staff that the symptoms and loss of function were variable in both time and space. They were often found to be most severe when parents were present and least severe when the children felt they were unobserved. Patients were able to use muscle groups for one action that they were unable to use for another. It is therefore not surprising that it has been debated as to whether the pathology of the illness lies in the muscle or moral fibre of the individual.

Q2. What do you know about the aetiological theories of chronic fatigue syndrome?

The reasons given for why some patients experience chronic fatigue are complex and probably multifactorial. The hypothesis is that the 'normal' sensation of fatigue experienced during a transient organic illness, such as a viral infection, is maintained by a variety of possible factors which may be psychological (premorbid personality, low self-esteem, psychiatric illness, e.g. depression and previous experience of illness) or social (family, school or peer-related problems). A common finding appears to be a perception of the child's under-achievement either by the individual him/herself or by his/her parents. The role of depression is uncertain but probably important in paediatric chronic fatigue syndrome.

The concept of 'abnormal illness behaviour' has been used to describe a variety of reactions, including chronic fatigue syndrome, which may present in the middle ground between medicine and psychiatry where physical complaints do not appear to have an obvious organic basis. School refusal is another important concept which itself may be a symptom of chronic fatigue syndrome. Here there is often separation anxiety which may be as pronounced in the mother as it is in the child. In some cases it is felt that parents are so prominent in the aetiology of this disorder that 'myalgic encephalomyelitis by proxy' as a possible variant of 'Munchausen syndrome by proxy' has been described. These parents may become inadvertently so involved in their child's illness as to perpetuate it and will often express exasperation in the medical profession's apparent 'incompetence' in understanding or managing the condition. They may then seek alternative treatments such as complex diets.

From the 'organic' side of the fence, various virions have generally been the proposed culprits. Herpes group viruses (in particular Epstein-Barr virus) and enteroviruses (in particular coxsackie B) have been implicated but despite investigation, no causal relationship has ever been confirmed. Indeed, despite the lay-press views to the contrary, adult studies have generally refuted the claim that the syndrome is caused by persistent viral infection following an attack of glandular fever.

Q3. OK, I'll stop you there. How severe is this illness?

The bottom-line is that it is very variable. Some children have prominent symptoms of fatigue and fatiguability but are still able to continue with some of their normal day. Many have periods where they have to withdraw from their normal routine, including becoming essentially bed-bound, although such episodes are usually transient and amenable to rehabilitation. However, Sidebotham et al (1992) have described very severe refractory cases in adolescents with prolonged episodes of apparent paralysis.

Q4. Briefly outline how you would manage a child with this syndrome.

I feel that multidisciplinary management is ideal, such as the joint paediatric–psychiatric approach outlined by Dr Vereker. An important member of this team is the GP who may have vital knowledge of the child's family dynamics and may also be the best person to take on the difficult process of engaging the patient and the family in the treatment (the so-called 'therapeutic alliance'). In addition, the psychiatrist in the team will be able to identify and instigate specific treatment if there is co-existing mental illness such as depression.

Although periods of rest are important, I would favour a programme of active rehabilitation, possibly with defined and agreed steps so that everyone concerned can work towards goals. Active rehabilitation can involve an outwardly physical approach with graded exercise supervised by another member of the team, the paediatric physiotherapist. This will often involve admission to hospital in which case the hospital teacher is another vital member so that the degree of impairment of personal and social development is minimised.

Above all, I would attempt to promote an atmosphere of optimism and try to ensure that the child is allowed to recover with honour, if necessary by focusing on the physical manifestations of his/her illness.

Tips

■ This question provides good ground on which to demonstrate that you have a gentle, caring approach and have built up experience of dealing with the 'whole patient' in your paediatric practice.

■ For situations like this where the management can be a little nebulous, it is useful to have in your mind a series of steps or points (as shown) which you can highlight in your response and use to structure your answer.

REFERENCES

Sidebotham P D et al 1994 Refractory chronic fatigue syndrome in adolescence. Case report. Br J Hosp Med 51: 110–112

Vereker M I 1992 Chronic fatigue syndrome; a joint paediatric-psychiatric approach. Arch Dis Child 67: 550–557

Hyperactivity

Q1. A mother comes to clinic with her 5-year-old son. She has seen a television programme about hyperactivity and believes her son is 'suffering' from this. How would you advise this mother?

First, I would like to explain what I understand by hyperactivity. Variously described as attention deficit hyperactivity disorder (ADHD), minimal brain dysfunction and hyperkinetic syndrome, it is severe, pervasive (i.e. present in all situations), impulsive behaviour, distractibility and poor attention span. Other features include aggressive behaviour with marked mood swings, low intelligence, learning difficulties, speech problems and poor sleep. To be differentiated from conduct and anxiety disorders, it has a prevalence of ~1 in 1000 in the UK, whereas in America estimates are much higher. Whether this is a true reflection of prevalence, rather than wider criteria for making the diagnosis, is difficult to answer. Male to female ratio is at least 3:1 and onset occurs before the age of 7.

From the mother I would like to know exactly what she understands by hyperactivity and why she believes that her son has it. Before she saw the television programme, did she have any concerns about her son's behaviour? Is she comparing her child's behaviour with that of a sibling or peers and has anyone else ever felt that there were problems (i.e. school, grandparents, family doctor)? Does she believe that there are reasons for her son's problems (e.g. food additives, birth trauma) and what measures has she tried to solve the problem (e.g. dietary manipulation, psychiatric input, drug therapy)? In the history taking, it is important to ask specifically about the birth and the neonatal period, developmental milestones, early behaviour and the temperament of the child, and family history. At what age did the family first think there was a problem, e.g. birth of a sibling, the start of nursery or school, the loss of a parent through death or divorce? It is important to exclude those children with age-appropriate behaviour and attention whose home or school are intolerant of normal childhood curiosity and activity. With the parents' consent, it would be worthwhile obtaining information from the child's school teacher about behaviour. Past medical history may reveal a history of breath-holding attacks, temper tantrums, encopresis, etc.

Some papers report a high incidence of soft neurological signs in ADHD and my examination would look particularly for these (mixed hand preference, poor hand–eye coordination, poor balance). Whilst talking through the history with the mother, I would assess child–parent interaction and look at the child's play activity. In particular, I would see if the child was able to concentrate on carrying out a particular task to its conclusion, e.g. drawing a picture or reading a story, although it must be borne in mind that hyperactive children can suppress characteristic behaviour in a structured situation such as the clinic. A child may not do as he/she is told because he/she cannot hear properly and I would therefore make an assessment of this.

Parents may expect answers and solutions from the initial consultation because you are the last hope! Athough time is short in outpatients, sympathy is essential and explanations about the diagnosis and treatment useful. Involvement of other specialties for assessment may be necessary, e.g. occupational therapy, physiotherapy, speech therapy, child psychiatry, and investigations may be indicated (thyroid function tests, EEG).

Q2. What treatment modalities are there for hyperactivity?

There are three broad categories:

1. *Behavioural therapies.* Both individual and family therapy may be warranted. The child needs to be given a structured daily routine for which compliance receives praise and rewards. Rules are made which tell the child what is right and what is wrong and transgressions result in deprivation rather than punishmnent. A period of time should be set aside each day when the child is allowed relaxation, but this should not be before bedtime. If disruption of the classroom is occurring, then individual lessons may be required — close communication and cooperation with the school is important.

2. *Drug therapies.* Central nervous stimulants such as amphetamines have been used in hyperactivity, but this is not first-line management. Long-term use can result in growth retardation and drug-free periods, e.g. school holidays, are necessary.

3. *Dietary manipulation.* This is an area of great controversy — anecdotal cases of dramatic improvement on dietary manipulation abound, especially in the media. 'E' numbers, e.g. tartrazine E102, sunset yellow E110 and benzoate E210-219, are particularly incriminated. There is no substantial evidence suggesting the efficacy of dietary manipulation and it most certainly can do some harm. If the family is adamant that certain foods are implicated, then dietary supervision with a specialist dietician is an acceptable approach.

Encopresis

Q. What is encopresis and how is it managed?

Encopresis is defined as 'faecal incontinence not due to organic defect, but most commonly a result of faulty toilet training, mental retardation, or regression'. More simply, it can be described as the passage of normal stools in inappropriate places after bowel control should have been established. It suggests major psychological abnormality and requires the joint care of paediatricians and clinical psychologist/psychiatrist. It probably accounts for <1% of children with soiling if the rigid definition of faecal incontinence without megarectum or impaction is taken.

Very often, however, encopresis is the label given to children with abnormal defaecation secondary to constipation. Once disimpaction has occurred and the child is passing soft stools, a pattern of regular bowel movement must be learnt. This is best achieved by sitting the child on the toilet for 5–10 minutes after meals, e.g. breakfast and dinner. The child requires encouragement and reward for first of all sitting on the toilet and then for passing a stool whilst on the toilet. Sitting on the toilet should never be a punishment but something that is routine and non-frightening. These children and their parents very often require long-term input from psychologists, in combination with appropriate medical treatment; otherwise family breakdown and long-term harm to the family may ensue.

Enuresis

Q1. A GP refers a 7-year-old boy who is bedwetting. You are seeing him for the first time with his parents in your outpatient clinic. How would you proceed?

Most children achieve control of bladder function by day by the age of 2–3 years and by night by 3–4 years. Enuresis is defined as uncontrolled micturition in children beyond a defined age (usually 4 years) and may be divided into primary (bladder control has never been achieved) or secondary (bladder control has been achieved and then lost) and day-time enuresis and/or night-time enuresis.

Dryness is a natural development which, like walking, emerges at an age determined by both genetic and environmental (including training) factors. Certain epidemiological facts are interesting and I would remind myself of these before I start any complicated management regimens.

— 15% of 5 year olds and 7% of 10 year olds wet the bed
— 1% of boys and 0.5% of girls are still bedwetting at 14 years
— bedwetting is commoner in boys than girls (possibly because a boy's bladder capacity is smaller)
— bedwetting is commoner in social classes 4 and 5 and in overcrowded homes
— there is a strong familial tendency with 70% having a first-degree relative with a history of enuresis
— there is an association with delayed speech development
— most children are psychologically normal
— treatment is rarely justified before 5–6 years.

Enuresis is a common problem and in many instances, after a brief initial assessment, an enuresis management programme can be discussed with the parents. I would, however, consider that I have two major responsibilities before I can safely do this, first to exclude an organic cause and second to exclude a serious psychological cause.

Organic causes are more likely if enuresis is secondary or day-time. Possible causes include UTI (6% of enuretic girls are found to have a UTI compared to 1.5% of non-enuretic girls), constipation, structural abnormality of the urinary tract (e.g. posterior urethral valves), neurological disease (such as mental handicap or spina bifida) or diabetes (mellitus or insipidus). Psychological causes are physical or sexual abuse or emotional deprivation.

I would take a history paying particular attention to:

— ever dry (primary or secondary)?
— day-time or night-time?

— age when parents and sibs achieved dryness?
— how often and to what extent is it a problem?
— general milestones?
— symptoms of neurological disease (weakness, difficulty walking)
— dribbling incontinence (always pathological)?
— polydipsia, polyuria, urgency, dysuria, haematuria?
— associated encopresis? (This small group of children are usually suffering from serious psychological or neurological illness)
— site and condition of toilet!
— related to school, birth of sibling, peer problems or bereavement?
— any other problems at home (marital, etc.)?
— parents' and the child's reaction to the 'accidents'?

I would then examine the child bearing in mind the possible organic and psychological causes and therefore paying particular attention to the abdomen, external genitalia, anal region (including perineal sensation — saddle-distribution loss suggests a sacral cord lesion), the spine and lower-limb neurology.

In most situations it will be clear from the consultation and observation of the family dynamics if a serious psychological cause is present. In the few circumstances when a sixth-sense tells me that things may be seriously amiss at home and that this may be a 'cry for help', I have often found that finding an excuse to interview either the child or one of the parents alone or contacting the GP or health visitor to be helpful. I would also contact social services to see if the child is on the 'at-risk' register.

My only initial investigations, unless I seriously considered an organic diagnosis, would be urinalysis and urine microscopy and culture.

Q2. Let's assume the boy has primary day-time enuresis and you have excluded an organic or serious psychological cause for his problem. Outline a plan of management.

I would explain carefully, in simple language, the process of achieving dryness to both the parents and the child reassuring all of them that this problem is both very common and likely to be outgrown. Sometimes I use simple diagrams and I would reiterate that the child has no physical or mental disease. I have often found that a sympathetic, confident and, above all, enthusiastic approach will pay dividends in treatment success.

In practice, simple measures will often already have been attempted by the child's GP and the reason for referral is perceived treatment failure, usually by the parents. In this situation, I would once again reassure them that the problem is very common, if necessary by quoting some of the figures I have already mentioned. Patience is truly a virtue when it comes to dealing with enuresis.

In the first instance, I would suggest that the parents keep a diary and reward good nights and ignore rather than punish bad ones. The idea of rewarding behaviour can be extended to the use of 'star charts' (or any emblem that the child likes — an enquiry about hobbies may be useful). A chart with a given number of stars could be further rewarded by a toy, for example. The star-chart method is particularly dependant on a confident, enthusiastic approach by the paediatrician and I would attempt to make both the boy and his parents feel part of a 'management team'. I would also organise a 2-week follow-up appointment so that everyone is aware when progress is to be reviewed.

By far the most effective and specific treatment is *buzzer alarms* which can be used in suitably intelligent children from the age of 5 years. The principle is conditioned learning. The mechanism is triggered by urine on a special mat underneath the child which sets off a buzzer. The boy should sleep without pyjamas so that the first drops of urine actuate the alarm. The alarm should be arranged so that he has to get out of bed to turn it of and he will then go to the toilet. The wet patches should get smaller and smaller as the boy is awakened earlier and earlier until he eventually wakes without actually voiding any urine or sleeps through without needing to micturate. With this system, 85% of children will become dry within 4 months. I would recommend continuing treatment until the boy has been dry for at least 6 weeks. The relapse rate is low at 10% and this would spur me to look once again for an underlying physical or psychological cause.

Occasionally, if there is an important event looming, such as a school holiday or a stay with friends, or if the boy's mother is at the end of her tether, a temporary prescription of desmopressin, which is a vasopressin analogue, may be useful. This is administered as a single intranasal dose of 20–40 µg at bedtime and acts by concentrating the urine, therefore reducing the nocturnal urine output. Desmopressin will produce improvement in about 80% of children and is relatively free from side-effects. I would generally only use it as a 'crutch' on a short-term basis rather than as main therapy and it is not recommended for use in children with CF. I would now rarely if ever use tricyclics such as imipramine in view of their side-effects, especially in over-dosage.

In some situations, admission to hospital for interval training may be justified. This may be because children with nocturnal enuresis also tend to pass frequent small volumes of urine by day.

School non-attendance

Q1. What do you know about children who fail to attend school?

This is a complex problem and I think the most important fact for a paediatrician to realise is that it is not a single diagnosis but rather a symptom of a number of possible problems. I would divide these into four main categories:

1. *Truancy* may be defined as school non-attendance as a manifestation of an underlying conduct disorder and is unfortunately one of the commonest reasons. It is vital that it is differentiated from school refusal.

Truancy tends to occur in older age groups (>8 years) and is associated with other anti-social behaviours such as delinquency and markers of social deprivation. Truants tend to stay away from home as well as from school and escape from a world of failure by finding a fantasy life of cinema, arcade games and football.

2. *School refusal* is non-attendance as a manifestation of an underlying neurotic illness.

School refusal may affect younger children (age 5 years and over) and represents a manifestation of either separation anxiety (fear of being away from parents) or school phobia (irrational fear of school). The former is worse on leaving home whereas the latter is worse on arriving at school. Unlike truants these children stay at home.

The neurotic reaction may be triggered by major psychological stress such as a bereavement or accident within the family and there are often associated psychosomatic symptoms such as headache or abdominal pain.

Other distinguishing features are:

	School refusal	*Truancy*
Previous attendance	Good	Poor
Personality	Conscientious, 'model' pupil High standards May be a loner	Rebellious Non-academic Mixes with other rebellious pupils
Family	Higher social classes Small family size May collude with the child to worsen attendance	Lower social classes Large family size Often unaware of the the non-attendance May be unconcerned

3. *Genuine reasons* for non-attendance. These include bullying or perceived

under-achievement or difficulty with certain teachers or lessons, such as 'games' or undiagnosed organic illness.

4. Occasionally, *parents* deliberately keep their children at home for a variety of reasons.

Therefore if faced with this problem, I would make a thorough evaluation so that I could instigate appropriate management. This would depend largely on a careful history from parents and child and observation of the family dynamics, backed up if necessary by discussion with the GP or teacher.

Occasionally, the history may point to underlying problems which make school a difficult place for the child, such as undiagnosed asthma, hearing loss, dyslexia or learning difficulties. Examination of the child will merely be to exclude any physical basis for the problem or any psychosomatic symptoms.

Q2. OK, briefly tell me how you would manage truancy or school refusal.

I will first deal with *school refusal*. Because of the nature of the problem and the usually favourable pre-morbid characteristics of these children, the prognosis is usually excellent. The key to school refusal is an early return to school. I would therefore counsel both parents and child and then set a definite date for return to school. I would collaborate with the teachers and sometimes the GP; in most cases, the services of a psychologist are not required. An Education Welfare Officer may, however, be able discretely to supervise the return. In situations where I feel that the parents are closely bound-up in the problem (sometimes to the extent where they may be perpetuating it), family therapy may be indicated.

Truancy is a far more difficult issue as it is so closely linked with numerous other social problems and the prognosis is generally poor. It requires a 'comprehensive management package' enlisting all relevant professionals. In particular, Social Services may be required. However, many of these children continue to display conduct disorders and not infrequently end up committing more serious offenses.

Eating disorders

Q. What do you know about anorexia nervosa?

Anorexia nervosa is the commonest eating disorder in adolescence. There has been an increase in incidence in recent years. It is ten times more common in girls than boys, but is otherwise similar in nature between the sexes. Prepubertal onset is rare, but when it occurs there is often a delay in diagnosis. Awareness of eating disorders among physicians appears to be limited and there is often delay between parents first seeking advice and referral to psychiatric services. This delay causes the disorder to become more entrenched and may therefore be more difficult to treat. A shorter history of illness before treatment has been found to be a good predictor of outcome.

Anorexia nervosa is characterised by a dread of fatness. The patient is convinced that she is too large and this perception remains even when she is severely emaciated. The disorder starts with a reduction diet in a girl who may have been teased about being overweight. Most adolescents who diet will not progress to anorexia and there may be an underlying difference in premorbid personality, with anorexics tending to have a pattern of dependence, compliance and perfectionism. There are signs of an obsessional compulsive disorder as the anorexic girl is often an expert on the calorific content of foods and may develop eating rituals. The girl may also have depressive symptoms with a low self-esteem, mood swings and restricted interests

Weight loss is achieved not only by dieting, but also rigorous exercise, abuse of laxatives and diuretics and vomiting. Binge eating and purging may be the next step, but bulimic features are infrequent in adolescent anorexics. The diagnosis of anorexia is classified as weight loss of 15% below that expected for age and height. It is also associated with physical characteristics due to starvation, which include amenorrhoea, bradycardia, hypothermia and electrolyte disturbances.

It is important to exclude medical illnesses, such as inflammatory bowel disease, diabetes mellitus and hyperthyroidism. These children lack the psychological features of anorexia. Assessment should include analysis of symptoms and significant life events prior to food refusal. Thoughts and attitudes to eating and weight should be explored. It may be found that the patient is fearful of becoming physically and emotionally mature. They also feel a lack of control over their lives and seek to correct this by strict control over their body and its functions.

Anorexia nervosa may become chronic in about 20% of patients, so intensive professional intervention should be offered at an early stage. It is sometimes managed on an outpatient basis if the family is supportive and the girl is highly motivated and cooperative. However, severe emaciation and family conflict would be criteria in favour of inpatient treatment. The major goal of treatment is weight gain. This should be done gradually with frequent small meals. The involvement of a dietician is helpful. In rare cases intravenous or nasogastric tube feeds may be life-saving, but should be avoided if possible to prevent disturbance of the staff–patient relationship. A member of staff should be present during meals.

Some patients benefit from individual psychotherapy, while others improve with family therapy. Behavioural therapy with a cognitive approach is frequently helpful, making use of positive and negative reinforcement, e.g. bed rest and seclusion if the anorexic will not cooperate with the regimen and visiting privileges if weight gain is achieved.

A multifaceted treatment programme is therefore required to improve the outcome of anorexia. Weight gain is achieved in about 60% of anorexics, but eating behaviour returns to normal in only 40%. Favourable prognostic factors include: early age at onset; conflict-free parent–child relationship; short interval between onset of symptoms and treatment intervention; short duration of inpatient treatment and high level of education.

In conclusion, anorexia nervosa is a disorder which is most common in adolescence, but presents late and may follow a chronic course if intervention is delayed.

Factitious illness

Q1. When would you suspect factitious illness in a child?

Factitious illness occurs when stories of illness are invented with the result that unnecessary investigation or treatment is undertaken.

In an older child, non-specific symptoms, such as headache or abdominal pain, which persist despite adequate doses of analgesia, may be suggestive of factitious illness. Typically, these children will miss school frequently. If admitted to hospital for assessment, they often have severe symptoms during the ward round but participate fully in ward activities for the rest of the day. Adolescents may also present with vomiting or diarrhoea, which they induce, and even haematuria, by the addition of blood to their urine specimens. These children are difficult to manage and unlikely to admit to their deception on direct confrontation. Their illness may be a way of expressing a need for concern and affection from their carers.

Factitious illness in a younger child is a form of abuse, which may pass unnoticed. It tends to be perpetrated by the mother, but it could be any carer closely associated with the child. Again it is usually common problems which present, e.g. vomiting, which is mechanically or chemically induced; seizures, which may be induced by suffocation; fever, by warming the thermometer or altering the charts; or rashes, made by scratching the skin surface.

Warning signs of factitious illness are:

— previous unexpected/unexplained sibling death
— previous non-accidental injury
— multiple illnesses in the family
— no effective or tolerated treatment
— mother always present when symptoms occur
— mother not as concerned as one would expect

Mothers of these children are often quite dominant and intelligent. They may admit to difficult childhoods and may also have unusual or unexplained illnesses themselves. They may previously have been nurses. They fit well into the ward environment and may be enthusiastic ward fundraisers.

Finally, factitious illness may occur in a third group of children. These usually have illnesses which could be described as fashionable, such as food allergy causing behavioural problems and hyperactivity or myalgic encephalomyelitis. It is usually an illness for which there is no diagnostic test, but the child will have seen many physicians and alternative practitioners in search of a cure. The mother and child both believe that it is a rare or special kind of illness to an almost delusional extent. They may produce newspaper articles to defend their case and will be very angry with the doctor who suggests that these symptoms may not be genuine. The child may himself realise that this is the case, but is in a difficult conspiracy with his/her mother due to a fear that exposure will cause rejection from the family. It is very difficult to challenge this belief system and, unless the child is malnourished due to dietary restrictions, when involvement of social services is warranted, intervention is likely to provoke the family to move on to the next practitioner.

It is important to recognise factitious illness. In the younger child, it is possible to prevent serious morbidity and mortality. In the older child, careful intervention may prevent a life-long career in factitious illness behaviour.

REFERENCE

Meadow R 1985 Management of Munchausen syndrome by proxy. Arch Dis Child 60: 385–393

Immunisation

Q1. How are vaccines classified?

The major classification is into *active* and *passive*. Active immunisation implies that 'activity' is evoked in the body to produce the immunity. This activity is stimulation of the immune system which therefore means that there is a delay before the protective effect is established. This is usually humoral or antibody mediated and therefore a successful response can be detected by laboratory serological testing. (BCG vaccine promotes cell-mediated immunity which is demonstrated by a positive tuberculin skin test.)

Passive immunisation implies that the body is a 'passive' bystander in the vaccination process as human immunoglobulin is injected. The protection afforded is immediate but lasts for only a few weeks.

Q2. Name some active vaccines.

Active vaccines may be killed organisms, live attenuated organisms or toxoids.

1. The main *killed* vaccines (heat or chemical inactivation) are:

    — Pertussis
    — Haemophilus (Hib)
    — Influenza
    — Typhoid/paratyphoid
    — Cholera
    — Rabies
    — Polio-inactivated (Salk)
    — Hepatitis B
    — Meningococcal — only against serotypes A and C
    — Pneumococcal

2. The main *live attenuated* vaccines are:

    — BCG
    — Rubella
    — Mumps
    — Measles
    — Polio-live (Sabin)
    — Yellow fever

3. The main *toxoids* are tetanus and diphtheria.

Q3. Tell me about passive vaccines.

Passive vaccines involve the administration of 'pre-made' human immunoglobulin which therefore gives immediate protection though only for a few weeks. There are of two types, pooled or specific.

Pooled immunoglobulin (human normal immunoglobulin or HNIG) is obtained from several normal individuals (who are HIV and HBV negative). The principle is that certain diseases have a relatively high prevalence in the community so that a reasonable number of the donors will have appropriate antibodies. HNIG is mainly used to give immediate protection against hepatitis A and is used for close contacts of all ages and also for travellers to all countries outside Northern Europe, Northern America, Australia and New Zealand.

HNIG also contains antibody to measles, varicella and other viruses which are currently prevalent in the population. It is not, however, recommended for the prevention of mumps or rubella. It may interfere with the immune response to live virus vaccines which should be given at least 3 weeks before or 3 months after an injection of HNIG.

Specific human immunoglobulin is available against chicken pox, hepatitis B, tetanus and rabies.

Q4. Remind my colleague and me about the current immunisation schedule.

1. *DPT, polio* and *Hib vaccine* is administered to all infants three times at 2, 3 and 4 months and this is known as the 'primary course'.
2. *MMR* is given to all children between 12 and 18 months of age. For those who for whatever reason have missed the routine administration, it can be given at any age over 12 months.
3. A booster of *DT* and *polio* is given to all children between 4 and 5 years.
4. A further *rubella vaccination* is administered to girls only, aged between 10 and 14 years (before their reproductive years).
5. A further booster of *tetanus* and *polio* is given to all children between 15 and 18 years.
6. The school nurse will also *tuberculin skin test* or Heaf test all school children aged between 10 and 14 years and BCG is administered to those without protection (never to individuals who show a positive reaction to tuberculoprotein). There should be an interval of 3 weeks between BCG and rubella or any other live vaccine administration.
7. In addition, at birth, BCG is given to all high-risk children, namely Asian children and where there is TB in a close contact. *Hepatitis B-killed vaccine* is given at birth to babies of high-risk mothers, especially if the mother is HB_eAg positive and HB_eAb negative (anti-HB_e negative).

Q5. You mentioned Hib vaccine. Tell me about this programme.

Since 1st October 1992, the routine UK primary immunisation schedule for infants has included vaccination against *Haemophilus influenzae type B* (Hib).

Invasive infection with *Haemophilus influenzae* includes meningitis, epiglottitis, septicaemia and septic arthritis/osteomyelitis. Young infants aged 6–12 months are at greatest risk, with haemophilus meningitis in this age group carrying a 5% mortality.

Almost all invasive infections are caused by encapsulated strains of *Haemophilus influenzae*, of which there are 6 serotypes, a–f. 84% of these serious infections are caused by type b. Non-encapsulated strains are not protected against by Hib vaccine but these generally cause mucosal infection only and rarely lead to serious disease.

In a UK study, three-stage Hib vaccination at 3, 5 and 9 months achievd protective levels of antibody in all of 103 infants (Tudor-Williams et al 1989). It has also been shown that a three-stage schedule administered earlier from 2 months of age with the 'primary course' (when the risk of Hib infection is rising sharply) is also effective; the antibody response is not significantly affected by placentally transferred maternal antibodies.

Large studies outside the UK have confirmed a rapid and profound reduction in the incidence of invasive Hib disease following the introduction of an immunisation programme. In Finland, the incidence of Hib meningitis in children aged 0–4 years has fallen from 30 per 100 000 to 0 in the first year of their vaccination programme in 1991.

As I mentioned earlier, together with DTP and polio, three-stage Hib vaccination is now part of the UK primary course at the ages of 2, 3 and 4 months. The Hib vaccine is given with a different syringe from DTP and into a different limb, so that local reactions can be recorded. Children aged 13 months or over (up to their 4th birthday) who have not been vaccinated need only a single dose to achieve protective antibody levels. Previous invasive Hib disease may not induce immunity in children under 2 years, so vaccination is still recommended. 20% of children given Hib will suffer mild local reactions. Other unwanted effects are no more likely than in those given DTP alone and so Hib vaccines have a good safety record.

Q6. Tell me about contraindications to immunisation.

In general terms, 'no child should be denied immunisation without serious thought as to the consequences both to the individual child and to the community' (Department of Health 1992).

The general contraindications are *intercurrent febrile illness*, when the administration should be merely delayed until the episode has resolved, and previous severe *general or local reaction* to the preceding dose. I would not consider a 'runny nose' without a pyrexia or systemic upset a reason to delay administration.

A severe general reaction is defined as fever of 39.5°C or higher within 48 hours of vaccination; anaphylaxis; laryngeal oedema; general collapse; prolonged unresponsiveness; prolonged inconsolable screaming, or convulsions within 72 hours. A severe local reaction is defined as 'an extensive area of redness and swelling which becomes indurated and involves most of the antero-lateral surface of the thigh or a major part of the circumference of the upper arm'.

Possible contraindications to *pertussis* immunisation have caused a great deal of concern and confusion in recent years. The current practice is that there is essentially no special contraindication to pertussis. Specifically, pertussis vaccination is not contraindicated in children with a personal or strong family history (including first-degree relative) of convulsions nor in those with documented cerebral damage (e.g. cerebral palsy or IVH). The only possible exception to this is in those with *progressive neurological disease* where it may be appropriate to delay pertussis immunisation to avoid the possibility of parents believing the vaccine is responsible for the illness. The current evidence suggests that 1 in 300 000 injections of pertussis vaccination may produce a neurological reaction within 7 days of immunisation of which only 2% per year in the UK are left with a permanent neurological defect.

Measles vaccination (including in MMR) is contraindicated if there is a history of an *anaphylactic reaction to eggs* (not just diarrhoea), in *immunocompromised* children or if there is known *allergy to neomycin*. Live polio (Sabin) vaccine should be delayed if these is *diarrhoea or vomiting* because of the likelihood of failure of uptake and is also contraindicated in *immunocompromised* children.

Q7. You mentioned immunocompromisation. Tell us a little more about the immunisation of immunosuppressed children.

Generally speaking immunosuppression contraindicates the administering of live vaccines. This includes high-dose corticosteroid (2 mg/kg/day for more than a week of prednisolone — where live vaccines are delayed until 3 months after treatment), leukaemia, lymphoma, chemotherapy or radiotherapy. In the latter two situations, vaccination should be delayed until at least 6 months after the chemo- or radiotherapy has been completed. These individuals may receive inactivated vaccines although these may be ineffective.

The exception to this is in the case of HIV-positive individuals with or without symptoms. These children should be given:

Live vaccines: Measles, mumps, rubella, polio
Inactivated vaccines: Pertussis, diphtheria, tetanus,
                      polio, typhoid, cholera, hepatitis B

HIV-positive individuals must *not*, however, receive BCG vaccine as there have been reports of BCG organism dissemination in such cases. Yellow fever vaccine should also not be given as there is insufficient data on its safety in HIV-positive individuals. Vaccine efficiency may, however, be reduced in these children and I would consider the use of normal immunoglobulin after exposure to measles.

Tips

■ Don't forget that the paediatric MRCP is the training qualification for community as well as hospital paediatricians — remember to cover primary care topics such as immunisation!

■ Keep up to date with changes to the usual schedule. In November 1994 there was a school-based national measles and rubella (MR vaccine) immunisation campaign for all children aged 5–16 years. The main purpose of the campaign was to prevent a measles epidemic predicted to occur in early 1995. In addition the campaign will improve the level of immunity against rubella which also appears to be falling off in young people. The provision of rubella in this campaign allowed discontinuation of the present school rubella immunisation programme for girls aged around 11 years from September 1994.

REFERENCES

Department of Health, Welsh Office, Scottish Home and Health Department 1992. Immunisation against infectious diseases. HMSO, London

Peltola H et al 1992 Rapid dispappearance of *Haemophilus influenzae* type b meningitis after routine childhood immunisation with conjugate vaccines. Lancet 340: 592-594

Tudor-Williams G et al 1989 *Haemophilus influenzae* type b conjugate vaccine trial in Oxford: implications for the United Kingdom. Arch Dis Child 64: 520–524

Walker D 1993 Immunisation — 125 years of progress. The Practitioner 237: 576–581

Accidents in childhood

Q1. What do you know about accidents in childhood?

Accidents are the main cause of death between the ages of 1 and 14 years, amounting to 700 deaths per year. They are also a source of considerable morbidity and emotional distress and every paediatrician should be aware of the scale of the problem. The best way to understand accidents in childhood is to consider the epidemiology:

1. *Leading causes of death by age group:*

4 weeks–1 year	Conditions arising in the perinatal period (46%)
	Congenital anomalies (16%)
1–4 years	Accidents (21%)
	Congenital anomalies (20%)
5–9 years	Accidents (34%)
	Cancer (22%)
10–14 years	Accidents (36%)
	Cancer (17%)

2. *Trends:* It is encouraging that child accident death rates have been decreasing from the late 1940s.

3. *Sex:* Boys have more accidents than girls with the ratio increasing with age.

4. *Social class:* Children in social classes IV and V have just over twice as many fatal accidents as those in I and II. The greatest differences relates to deaths from fire with a ratio of 5 in this category.

5. *Location of accidental deaths:*

	0–4 years	5–14 years
Home	55%	16%
Transport-related	33%	76%
Other	12%	8%

6. *Nature of fatal accidents.* In order (age 0–15 years) they are road traffic accidents (56%), fire, etc. (13%), drowning (10%), choking (4%), falls, mechanical suffocation, poisoning and electrocution.

The Government's White Paper 'The Health of the Nation' (1991) sets a target of reducing death rates for accidents among children aged 15 years and under by at least a third by the year 2005. This translates as a reduction from 6.5 to 4.5 or less per 100 000 population.

Most accidents stem from either ignorance or failure to implement what is known. Therefore, some authorities advocate the use of the term 'injuries' rather than 'accidents' which suggest they are not random but rather predictable events which can be prevented (Smith & Pless 1994).

Q2. OK, outline the processes by which we may achieve a reduction.

Prevention of childhood accidents should be of prime importance to all members of society, including health professionals. Possibilities for targeting prevention exist at a variety of levels:

1. *The Paediatrician.* Opportunistic education should be undertaken, including the use of leaflets and posters, etc. in clinics and on wards. Verbally endorsing these to parents is very important. Parents should be advised about the scale of the problem and the importance of preventive measures. Children have a great capacity for curiosity and may be blissfully unaware of hazards which may be obvious to the adult. Various aspects of accident safety can be covered:

— general care at home
— falls: stair and seating/surface safety
— accidental poisoning: use and storage of drugs and chemicals
— burns and scalds: use of electrical, heating and kitchen equipment.
— lacerations: use and storage of knives, etc.
— choking: care with certain foods (e.g. nuts) and small objects
— suffocation: care with polythene bags
— care at bathing times and with open water, e.g. ponds
— sibling protection: advise that older sibs can be unwittingly dangerous if not supervised
— pedestrian safety: e.g. 'the Green Cross Code'
— cycle safety: use of helmets
— car safety: encouraging the use of correct restraints

Other opportunities for the paediatrician include: secondary prevention, e.g. after a child is admitted with accidental poisoning, scalds, falls, etc; care with prescribing, e.g. avoiding tricyclics; teaching first-aid (this is not strictly accident prevention but should go hand-in-hand with it), e.g. resuscitation techniques, the various methods of dislodging an inhaled foreign body; safety in the hospital — the paediatrician should always be alert to the possible sources of danger to a child on the wards or in clinic; health education in schools; helping with/ organising campaigns; finally, a paediatrician could conduct local studies or audits of childhood accidents.

2. *The A&E department.* Casualty staff could become involved in many of the above (in particular in secondary prevention — 1 in 6 children are brought to an A&E department each year). The waiting areas can be utilised for the display of leaflets and posters.

3. *The GP and health visitor.* As well as all the above, accident prevention should be a central issue in child surveillance. Members of the primary health care team

should exploit the fact that they have more regular access to children and their parents. In addition, they also have a unique possibility to actually see parents and children at home and offer specific advice.

4. *Designers* could in theory drastically reduce the number and severity of many accidents both inside and outside the home although, in many cases, the increased cost of 'safe' designs has limited this aspect of prevention. Parents should be advised to look for safety markings (e.g. the kite mark).

Important 'objects' include:

— toys
— prams and chairs
— car seats and restraints
— drug and chemical containers
— household utilities, e.g. electrical goods, plugs, etc.
— fire retarding materials which do not emit toxic gases
— housing design including windows, staircases, etc.
— car and cycle design

5. *Town and highway planning*. This is another area with great potential which is again unfortunately limited by cost.

—, safer speed-retarding road layouts with greater visibility
— greater steps to separate children at play and cars
— illumination of roads
— siting and safety of cycleways, parks, etc.
— design of schools, playgrounds and swimming pools

6. *Campaigns and organisations*, e.g. television campaigns, the Royal Society for the Prevention of Accidents, accident prevention units, police (road safety officer), local programmes targeted at high-risk neighbourhoods.

7. *Legislation*. Although people consider some legislation to be an infringement on freedom, in some situations it has a vital role in accident prevention.

— vehicle and road safety, e.g. speed limits, alcohol limits, restraints in cars
— legislation relating to the materials used in the manufacture of furniture
— design of toys

8. *Information*. It is important that information on types of accidents, particularly from A&E departments and the Police is collated in order for areas needing improvement to be identified. Depending on the area, Accident Prevention Units or the local Family Health Service Authority (FHSA) may take part in local initiatives.

REFERENCE

Smith R, Pless I B 1994 Preventing injuries in childhood. Br Med J 308: 1312–1313

Sudden infant death syndrome

Q. A mother on the postnatal ward is concerned about the possibility of sudden infant death syndrome in her infant. What would be your advice to her and why?

I would initially examine the baby to reassure the mother that she has a healthy child. I would ask her what she already knows about the sudden infant death syndrome (SIDS), or cot death. I would specifically enquire about previous infants in the family who have suffered a cot death, since her fears may be due to a previous neonatal death.

I would check the weight of the infant, since there does seem to be a slight increase in risk in low birthweight infants. There is also a higher risk in multiple births. If all of these factors are negative, I would proceed to make practical suggestions based on research.

There seems to be no doubt that maternal smoking, both antenatally and postnatally, increases the risk of sudden infant death. The risk is dose dependant. I would strongly urge a smoking mother to give up and suggest that other household members should do so also.

Many retrospective studies have shown that sleeping position may be important and a prospective study has confirmed this. It has been found that more infants have died unexpectedly and without obvious cause when laid prone. Educating parents to lay their baby *supine* has been shown to reduce the rate of cot death. It has been suggested that the prone position, by keeping the face partially covered, may prevent the infant from regulating body temperature adequately. The increase in risk has not been shown to be due to airway obstruction.

Previously, most babies have slept on their fronts due to concern that the infant is at increased risk of aspiration of vomit or choking. However, this has not been proven. I would not recommend that a child be laid supine if there is a history of severe gastro-oesophageal reflux or in those with an obstructive airway problem, such as Pierre-Robin syndrome.

I would suggest to this mother that she lies the infant flat on his/her back to sleep. If the child will not settle in that position he/she can be nursed on his/her side with the lower arm in front of the body, so that he/she cannot roll to the prone position. I would advise against putting a rolled up sheet under the upper shoulder as this increases the risk of the child rolling on to his/her front.

A child over the age of about 5–6 months is capable of rolling onto his/her front. I would reassure the mother that when her child reaches this age the risk of SIDS is greatly reduced and she need not keep putting the child back into the supine position.

Studies have shown that infants who died of cot death have been at greater risk of *overheating*. This has been due to greater insulation of their clothing and bedding, as well as higher room heating, for a given ambient temperature. A normal infant should be able to regulate body temperature. In a febrile illness, the metabolic rate is higher and this may make temperature control more difficult. However, by definition the infant with SIDS should not have an underlying illness and it is not known what, apart from covering the face, is disturbing temperature regulation.

I would suggest to the mother that she should be careful not to overwrap the child, especially if he/she is unwell or feverish. The child's room should be 16–20°C. Bedding should not be excessive and should be arranged so that the child cannot slip below the covers. A hat is unnecessary indoors in an infant over a month of age.

If the mother is intending to *breast feed*, I would reinforce this idea strongly. Some research has suggested that breast feeding reduces the risk of SIDS. This view has not been backed up in all studies and may reflect the fact that the breast feeding population are those least likely to smoke.

Finally I would advise the mother to seek medical advice if the child seems at all unwell, as trivial illnesses in the infant may be more serious than they seem.

The mother may ask for an apnoea monitor. If there are no risk factors for SIDS, I would discourage her by explaining that there is no proof that the use of apnoea alarms reduces the incidence of cot death. If an apnoea alarm is indicated, e.g. if a previous sibling had a cot death and the parents are keen to have the alarm, I would teach them basic resuscitation.

Until the causes of sudden infant death syndrome are more precisely defined, these recommendations are the most practical in an attempt to reduce incidence.

Non-accidental injury

Q1. What injuries in a child would make you suspect non-accidental injury?

Non-accidental injury (NAI) is only one cause of child abuse, albeit the commonest (the others include emotional deprivation, sexual abuse, neglect and Munchausen syndrome by proxy). It accounts for ~100 deaths a year in the UK and many more serious permanent injuries.

Abused children may present in a number of different ways and in a variety of settings — recognition is rarely straight forward. As always, clear and accurate documentation (and if appropriate colour photography) of the injuries is essential, including a detailed history of how the injuries were obtained, preferably from more than one person. Social and family circumstances and past medical history must be obtained. Relevant details of history pointing towards a diagnosis of NAI include:

1. Delay in seeking medical help
2. Inadequate, unrealistic or inconsistent explanation of the injuries, e.g. a 1-month-old sustaining a spiral tibial fracture by rolling over in his/her cot
3. Inappropriate, indifferent or over-concerned attitude of carer
4. Accompanying adult is someone other than the parents and there is no good reason why a parent is not present
5. A history of previous injuries or attendance to casualty for the child or siblings, e.g. burns, scalds, ingestions, fractures
6. Accompanying person is unwilling to allow full examination of the child
7. Child or sibling is on the 'at risk' register

Features of the examination of importance include:

1. *Distribution and nature of soft issue injures*. Every mobile child has bruising of the shins but it would be worrying in a 2 month old. Similarly infants attempting to sit and stand may have bruising to the forehead but not in a 2 month old. It is extremely difficult for a child to bruise around the neck area as the head and shoulder protect this area very well. Bruising of different ages is of significance although it is extremely difficult to age bruises accurately and it is something that I cannot or would not do with any degree of certainty.

2. *Distribution and nature of fractures*. Fractures in under 1s are very rare and uncommon in under 3s. Greenstick fractures are much less sinister than spiral fractures of long bones. Metaphyseal chip/bucket handle fractures are highly suggestive of NAI.

3. *Highly suggestive injuries.* These include bite marks, cigarette burns, torn frenulum, immersion scalds to hands, feet and buttocks, subconjunctival haemorrhages, finger-tip bruises, demarcated bruises and abrasions caused by belts, shoes and the slapping hand of an adult.

Q2. OK, so you have a child that you suspect has NAI. How would you proceed?

As already mentioned, it is essential to have a detailed history from all parties with accurate documentation of all injuries sustained. The need for social service input is essential early on — a 24-hour emergency duty team are available and if prosecution is anticipated, then the child protection unit needs to be involved. If there is a possibility of child sexual abuse, then joint examination is required with the police surgeon and I would seek the advice of my consultant on call regarding procedure. Great emphasis is often placed on investigations with clotting studies and skeletal survey, but these are rarely contributory. The skeletal survey involves significant exposure to radiation and must not be undertaken lightly. If it is deemed necessary, it should be carried out during 'working hours' when specialised paediatric radiographers are available. Hospital is not a suitable place for a child with NAI unless medically unfit to be discharged and very often a child can be safely placed at home, providing the perpetrator is not present. Alternatively, social services may provide emergency foster carers for such eventualities.

My role would be to document the injuries and state whether the explanation given is satisfactory, rather than organise placement of the child. Almost certainly, a case conference will be convened in the near future and worthwhile input by the hospital paediatrician justifies attendance whenever possible.

Perianal redness

Q. What thoughts run through your mind when you see a child with perianal redness?

Possible diagnoses include:

— napkin dermatitis
— candidiasis
— seborrhoeic dermatitis
— psoriasis
— drug rash
— streptococcal dermatitis
— thread worm infestation
— Crohn's disease
— child sexual abuse

The likelihood of each of these is dependent upon the age of the child, associated symptoms and signs, previous treatment and social circumstances.

1. *Napkin dermatitis.* In nappy-wearing infants and children, this is a red raw appearance confined to the nappy area with sparing of the inguinal folds. Treatment requires regular nappy changes (or better still, leaving the nappy off altogether) and protected barrier ointment (zinc, castor oil); 1% hydrocortisone cream will clear up the rash very quickly

2. *Candidiasis.* If napkin dermatitis has been present for longer than a few days, fungal infection is highly likely. The rash is beefy red and scaly with discrete satellite lesions. Treatment with topical and oral antifungals ± hydrocortisone will be very effective.

3. *Seborrhaeic dermatitis.* Yellowish greasy scales sometimes on an erythematous background seen on the head and face of babies, but it can involve the napkin area where scaling may be absent. Treatment is simple emollients, liquid paraffin or salicylic acid preparations for the cradle cap and emollients and exposure to the nappy area.

4. *Psoriasis.* Uncommon in childhood and usually with a family history. Pitting of the nails and scalp involvement must be looked for. Guttate psoriasis is usually preceded by a viral URTI and settles spontaneously. Plaque psoriasis requires topical tar preparations, salicylic acid, oral retinoids, PUVA with cytotoxics and intra-lesional steroids for more severe cases.

5. *Drug rash.* Virtually any drug can result in an idiosyncratic reaction and if suspected the drug should be stopped.

6. *Streptococcal perianal dermatitis*. Characterised by an erythematous, confluent, moist pruritic eruption associated with painful defaecation and blood-streaked stools. Diagnosis is made by culture of a swab of the perianal region and treatment is with oral penicillin or erythromycin.

7. *Thread worm infestation*. *Enterobius vermicularis* infestation is common in young school children as high as 40–50% in 5–6 years olds. Night-time migration of the gravid female from the colon to the anal margin where she deposits her eggs results in pruritus, and secondary bacterial infection is possible. Diagnosis by transparent adhesion tape applied to the perianal skin in the morning, followed by microscopy, is the most successful method. Treatment is with mebendazole.

8. *Crohn's disease*. Perianal disease may be the first manifestation of Crohn's disease in children. Other signs and symptoms must be looked for including growth failure, abdominal pain, oral aphthous ulceration, diarrhoea and all the extra-intestinal manifestations.

9. *Child sexual abuse*. Anal fissuring can also indicate sexual abuse. Herpes simplex virus II infection and other sexually transmitted diseases may be present. If suspected, involvement of social services and the police is essential.

Teenage smoking

Q1. What do you know about teenagers and smoking?

Smoking is a destructive habit which is known to predispose to numerous diseases, including cancers (bronchus, cervix, oesophagus, bladder), chronic lung disease, vascular diseases and fetal diseases from maternal smoking. In addition, there is increasing evidence that smoking is a significant risk factor for the later development of osteoporosis (Valimaki et al 1994). The earlier an individual begins to smoke, the greater the risk of many of these.

It is also anti-social; the risks of passive smoking become increasingly recognised. Passive childhood smoking is known to be linked with the development of respiratory diseases.

It is therefore unfortunate that unlike the trend in adults, childhood smoking is increasing and girls appear to be more likely to smoke than boys. 10% of 11–15 year olds smoke regularly and among 15 year olds a staggering 1 in 4 smoke. Girls are likely to be strongly influenced by their mother and their closest friend; boys by peers.

Q2. OK, What are the possible methods by which we could reduce smoking in childhood?

This is a difficult problem since there is resistance not only from the participants (and adolescents are a group particularly resistant to health education) but also from a variety of ill-defined politically related sources. Despite the Government's impressive 'Health of the Nation' suggested targets for smoking reduction, the immense revenues from tobacco taxes tend to soften the implementation of any real changes in policy.

1. *Hospital staff*. Health education, both passive (in the form of posters and leaflets) and active (directed at parent and child), may have some effect.

2. *GPs and health visitors*. As above, but also:
   — 'well adolescent' clinics. There is debate about the value of clinics for healthy teenagers. The 'inverse care law' applies, i.e. the ones who are likely to attend least tend to be those who are most in need and vice versa. However, the small proportion of teenagers who do attend may be encouraged either to stop smoking or not to start. In addition, educated motivated teenagers may exert positive peer pressure on 'offenders'
   — offering interviews. As with the general management of 'difficult adolescents', offering interviews to teenagers who are known to smoke

may allow them to talk about any underlying problems and also provide an opportunity for health education.

3. *Advertising*. There is evidence that adolescents are very susceptible to advertising by tobacco companies and will buy certain brands and not just the cheapest cigarettes. There is also no doubt that some advertising campaigns deliberately or otherwise appeal directly to children.

4. *Schools*. Health education at an early age may have preventive value. Ideally, this should be 'user-directed' and not conducted by someone who is perceived as an aloof teacher.

5. *Legislation*. Stricter control of the portrayed image of cigarettes would definitely have a bearing on the prevalence of teenage smoking. This could cover various areas such as: general tobacco advertising, television image, availability, cigarette-like sweets.

It is important that health workers continue to apply pressure on the Government to tighten legislation relating to tobacco advertising. The ideal would be a complete ban on advertising and exorbitant taxes on cigarettes.

REFERENCE

Valimaki M et al 1994 Exercise, smoking and calcium intake during adolescence and early adulthood as determinants of peak bone mass. Br Med J 309: 230–235

Confidentiality and the teenager

Q. I want you to imagine you are a Consultant Paediatrician and a girl of 13 has been admitted to your ward at 4 am with acute asthma. You see her on your morning wardround at which time she is still fairly wheezy but stable. You inform her that she is likely to be kept in hospital for a couple of days at which point she tells you that she is on the oral contraceptive pill and does not want her mother to be informed of this. What are your thoughts? Was her GP right to put her on the pill without her parents' consent? Does the girl have a right to prevent you from discussing this with her mother?

In this day and age, there are an increasing number of girls under the age of 16, and even as young as 13, on the pill. Adolescent contraception highlights many potential problems relating to confidentiality, conflict of interests and the underage teenager. The 1985 House of Lords' ruling by Lord Fraser in the Victoria Gillick case has established the legal position of doctors in respect of underage contraception and the principles within the statement have been used to guide practice in broader issues of teenage confidentiality. Basically, the ruling stated that it is not unlawful to provide contraceptive services to a girl under 16 as long as the girl can understand the advice given (including the potential risks); the doctor has attempted to persuade the girl to inform her parents; the girl is likely to begin or continue to have sexual intercourse even if contraception is not provided; her physical or mental health are likely to suffer if the services are not provided; and it is in the girl's best interest to provide contraceptive services without parental consent.

A subsequent guidance report entitled 'Confidentiality and People Under 16' issued jointly by various bodies, including the BMA and The Royal College of General Practitioners, essentially reiterates that the duty of confidentiality owed to a person under 16 is as great as that owed to any other person and that any competent young person, regardless of age, can independently seek medical advice and give valid consent to medical treatment.

Thus, providing the GP had satisfied him or herself of the points in the Fraser ruling, it is entirely reasonable that this girl was prescribed the pill without the knowledge of her mother. (Indeed, in Britain in 1988 there were approximately 9000 pregnancies to girls under 16, 53% of which were aborted. The Government's publication 'The Health of the Nation' sets a target of halving the pregnancy rate in the under 16s by the year 2000.) The girl has every right to insist that her confidentiality in this regard is maintained and steps should be taken to safeguard this, e.g. informing all staff who may have learned of her contraception of her wish that her mother is not made aware and the treatment chart is removed from her bedside.

Decisions must also be made as to whether to continue her on the pill whilst she is in hospital and there are obvious implications if she requires a course of broad-spectrum antibiotics.

Problems of adolescence

Q1. Tell me what you understand by the terms puberty and adolescence.

Puberty refers to the biological changes concerned with maturation of the older child into an adult with particular regard to sexual maturation. *Adolescence* refers to the psychological changes or new feelings around the pubertal period and to the individual's adjustment to them. The WHO defines adolescence as the period from 11 to 21 years.

Q2. What do you know of the psychology of adolescence?

Adolescence is a transition period in many aspects of the psychological development of a child and coincides with transitions in many other facets of his/her life. Of note is the fact that it usually also marks a period of transition for the parents, especially relating to loosening of protective bonds. Usually, these factors combine to result in a highly turbulent time for the family unit; however, this is not inevitable and cultural and environmental factors are of great importance in determining how the individuals handle and respond to this period.

Perhaps the two main aspects of adolescent development are the search for a sense of identity and independence and sexual maturation. The striving for a sense of identity goes hand in hand with the desire for independence and begins with the development of a questioning and even ambivalent attitude towards parents. Relationships can become increasingly strained and stresses can be placed on all elements of the family unit. Sometimes, teenagers rebel and deliberately 'go against the grain' with their parents and teachers and yet continue to ask themselves why they are behaving in this way. In contrast, peer relationships are largely uncritical as peers represent the focus for the intense dependency needs of early adolescence and are intrinsic to the formation of social identity. Opportunities for part-time work may be a symbol of the desire for financial or work independence as well as social independence.

The adolescent mind is also unsettled by the surge of sexual feelings and sexual experimentation which enhance the long established gender role and steadily, or unsteadily, lead the child towards his/her own sexual identity.

Careful handling of the adolescent phase by parents, if necessary with guidance, is essential to smoothing over these potentially unstable years and may also reduce the risk of harmful behaviour and psychiatric illness.

Q3. You mentioned careful handling of adolescent children by their parents. Do you know of any principles of management?

Perhaps the most important principle is to *treat* adolescents seriously but not to *take* them seriously, this being a self-protection policy as well as serving to minimise rebellious behaviour. The difficult adolescent should be thought of as a boat on a stormy sea and the parents as a lighthouse; the parents show the child 'direction' rather than journeying out to join them in the troubled waters. We also know that the hallmark of teenagers who do cope with this difficult period in their lives is high self-esteem and, as far as possible, parents should encourage this feeling in their children.

Q4. OK, what are the more serious problems of adolescence?

I would consider the more serious problems of adolescence under two main headings, *harmful behaviour* and *psychiatric illness*, although many cases fall into both categories.

From lifestyle surveys, we know that teenagers do feel responsible for their own health and do agree that good health is mainly due to sensible living. However, we also know that adolescents are at risk of harmful behaviour such as smoking, alcohol excess, substance abuse, criminal behaviour including vandalism, violence and 'joy-riding', unsafe sex and unwanted pregnancy.

The adolescent period is also prone to various psychiatric illnesses such as eating disorders (anorexia nervosa and bulimia nervosa), major 'neurotic' disorders such as obsessive neurosis and depressive illness and major 'psychotic' disorders such as manic depressive illness and schizophrenia.

Q5. Tell me about sexual behaviour in adolescents

Surveys have shown that 31% of under 16 year olds are sexually active and the trend is increasing. In addition, questionnaires reveal there are unmet needs amongst teenagers to discuss sexual development, sexually transmitted diseases (STD) and contraception. Although the majority of sexually active teenagers do have some experience of contraception, first intercourse and casual or unplanned encounters are likely to be unprotected. Sexually active teenagers are therefore particularly at risk of STDs and unwanted conception.

Q6. What do you know about teenage pregnancy?

Adolescent conception is an increasing problem, with rising conception rates in the under 16s. In 1990, 1% of 13–15-year-old girls became pregnant and about half of these resulted in abortion. The 'Health of the Nation' target is to reduce the rate of conception in the under 16s by at least 50% by the year 2000. Young people most at risk from pregnancy lack self esteem, show low educational achievement and are from an unhappy background such as broken families or being in care.

Pregnant teenagers suffer higher risk of antenatal and postnatal problems, including poor antenatal clinic attendance, pre-eclampsia, premature labour and postnatal depression. Rather surprisingly, the teenage intrapartum period is often problem free. Indeed they have been described as 'model labourers' as far as primigravidas go. Approximately one-third of teenage pregnancies end in legal abortion and at this age, 'would-be' mothers are particularly likely to experience severe emotional problems as a consequence.

The off-spring of pregnant teenagers have a higher rate of low birthweight, SIDS, NAI and developmental problems.

Informing parents of a non-organic diagnosis

Q. Imagine that for 2 months you have been looking after Stuart, an 8-year-old boy with a 6-month history of recurrent vomiting. You have seen him as both an inpatient and outpatient. You are confident that you have excluded an organic cause for his symptoms and feel that a variety of factors including family- and school-related stresses are contributing to his problem. Tell me how you would break this news to his parents and plan initial management.

This is an interesting problem and one which is frequently met in paediatrics. I have usually found it important to have an open and frank discussion at the outset so that both the parents and myself are aware of the situation from both sides and we can effectively plan Stuart's management. This would be an arranged meeting with both parents at a mutually convenient time. I would ensure I had enough time so as not to be hurried and I would take steps to prevent interruption, including freeing myself of my bleep. I would arrange a quiet room and preferably have a nurse present who has the trust of Stuart's parents.

Within the interview, I would assume an optimistic manner and use plain English, avoiding medical jargon. Hopefully I would already have the trust and confidence of the parents built up over the past 2 months. I would call the family by name and start by exploring their perception, beliefs and understanding regarding their son's illness and its causation. My aim would be to incorporate them into Stuart's management team.

I usually start the active phase of my interview by reassuring them that Stuart's problem is a common one and one which I have dealt with several times before. Next, I would remind them that I have now looked after their son for some time and explain carefully that I am confident that we have excluded any physical cause for the vomiting, if necessary by highlighting some of the investigations. It is important at this stage to explain that it is not unusual for this to be the case. Parents are usually relieved when I reiterate that their child does not have a serious, life-threatening illness such as cancer to account for symptoms. I would next explain that although we have not found a physical cause for this problem, the condition is still a very real one and, if necessary, I would offer a label such as 'chronic idiopathic vomiting'. I have found that parents often feel better if they have a 'label' upon which to focus their thoughts and this is also useful with respect to dealing with relatives, friends and school members to avoid talk of "he's that disturbed boy".

With severe somatic reactions, it is often beneficial from everyone's point of view to commence management in hospital and so, if the boy is not already an inpatient, I would explain why this may be necessary.

It is important to concentrate on what we *do know* and *can do* and so I would ensure that this forms the central part of my counselling. I would therefore explain that I have organised a 'treatment team' so we can help Stuart overcome this illness and *they* are an important part of this team. It is however important that neither Stuart nor his parents feel crowded, although it may be useful in individual cases for a variety of people to play a superficial role, including the child psychiatrist, dietician and teacher. I therefore usually focus upon one person primarily to effect the programme of management, e.g. a sympathetic paediatric-physiotherapist may be ideally suited to being acceptable to both the boy and his parents. I would explain that my management programme will involve graded steps which may take the form of exercises and that Mrs Jones, our physiotherapist, will be supervising these. The idea of this is based around the principle of distraction so that Stuart can find a way to re-enter his normal life without continued vomiting.

Tackling the precipitating reasons for Stuart's problem is usually more difficult and I have often found that the problems stem either from school or the family dynamics, or both. I would have normally spoken to the GP by this time and he or she will often be able both to identify and help manage specific family-related problems. Stuart or his teachers may well have already brought to my or his parents, attention school troubles and in some cases if these cannot be resolved, a change of school may be the easiest option.

Finally, I would ask the parents whether they had any questions and then arrange our next meeting to discuss how things are going and tackle any new problems. I would explain that I have discussed the situation fully with their GP and so if they have any new thoughts or questions in the mean time that they are welcome to contact either of us.

Tip

- A difficult question if you are not prepared for it! Try and demonstrate that you have dealt with this sort of problem and also show that you have a caring, gentle nature.

Children Act

Q. What are you able to tell me about the Children Act 1989?

Royal assent for the act was given on the 16th November 1989, but it was not fully implemented until October 1991. Essentially a document for the protection of children, it replaced the Children and Young Persons Act 1969. In essence its key message is to place the welfare of the child above all other considerations and to strike a balance between family independence and the protection of the child. The Act prevents the implementation of Court orders unless it contributes positively to the child's welfare. (A child is any individual under the age of 18.) Salient features of the Act include:

1. The child's welfare shall be the Court's paramount consideration. The Court should not make any order unless doing so would be better for the child than not doing so.
2. The prime responsibility for bringing up children should lie with the parents and responsibility replaces that of parental right.
3. Local authorities should provide, or cause to provide, supportive services to assist parents in bringing up their children.
4. Local authorities are required to take reasonable steps to identify children and families in need, these children being defined as:
   — a child unlikely to achieve or maintain, or have the opportunity of achieving or maintaining, a reasonable standard of health development without the provision of services by a local authority
   — a child whose health or development is likely to be significantly impaired or further impaired without the provision of such services
   — a child who is disabled
   Every local authority should open and maintain a register of children with disabilities.
5. Sensitivity to ethnic considerations in assessing the child's needs, in providing services and in communication of services available.
6. Working in partnership with parents, involving them in decision making and being more responsive and flexible to meet the needs of the child and family.

The Children Act 1989 provides a series of Orders for the protection of children who are 'at risk.'

1. Emergency protection order (EPO). This has replaced the Place of Safety Order. Any individual may apply to the Magistrate's Court for an EPO and parental responsibility is then transferred to this person. Maximum

duration is 8 days with possible extension by a further 7 days and an appeal can be made after 3 days.

2. Child Assessment Order. This enables proper assessment of a child, lasting up to a maximum of 7 days, but does not necessarily involve removal of the child from the family home and parental responsibility is not transferred from the parents.

3. Care and Supervision Orders. These enable children to be placed in the care of and under the supervision of a local authority respectively. Maximum duration for both is 8 weeks.

4. Police Protection provisions. Any police constable may take a child into police protection for up to 3 days without assuming parental responsibility.

Statementing

Q. What can you tell me about statementing?

According to the 1981 Education Act, which was updated in 1993, the local education authority must provide a statement for children with special educational needs in order that they may benefit fully from their education. The aim is for these children to have a broad and balanced education, ideally amongst their peers in mainstream schools.

The statement is made after assessment by interested parties and sets out the child's educational and non-educational needs. It declares the provision that should be made for the child and indicates when that need should be reviewed.

Many children have special educational needs, including those with chronic illnesses, e.g. a child with cystic fibrosis who has limited mobility and therefore needs lessons on the ground floor; a child with leukaemia who may miss a lot of school; or a child with epilepsy whose medication causes learning difficulties. However, statementing is most commonly used in those children with complex needs, e.g. the child with developmental delay, visual impairment and learning difficulties.

The statement should include all available information about the child, with the views of the parents and relevant professionals included. It must give a clear account of the services to be offered and be written in easily understood language.

There are various appendices to the statement, which include evidence from the parents and advice from the educational psychologist, teacher, community paediatrician, speech therapist, physiotherapist and occupational therapist where applicable. It will take into account whether the child needs one-to-one supervision, a quiet area to avoid distraction and group activity to help develop communication skills. The statement also suggests whether the child needs transport to school. The statement will name an appropriate school.

Early identification of these children is important so that adequate provision can be made at an early stage. The need for regular review should be included within the statement.

Disability living allowance

Q. What do you know about the disability living allowance?

The disability living allowance was introduced in 1992 to replace the attendance and mobility allowance. It was designed to help to cover the extra costs involved when a child is disabled. It consists of two parts:

1. *Care component*. A child is entitled to this if he requires 'substantially more care from another person than a child of the same age'. It has three rates and may be started from birth. It is further divided into:

   a) *Attention* — Which allows for help with normal bodily functions such as breathing, seeing, eating and communication. Encopresis and enuresis may qualify.

   b) *Supervision* — allows for the need to have a carer constantly present and ready to intervene to prevent danger.

The child's needs may be as a result of physical or mental disability, which need not be a chronic problem.

2. *Mobility allowance*. This has two rates and cannot be claimed before the age of 5. The higher rate is paid if the child is unable to walk, either due to physical impairment or because the behaviour is so unpredictable that a carer needs to be present physically to intervene to prevent injury. The lower rate applies to children who need more help than another child of the same age to be safe or to find their way around.

Help must be needed for a period of at least 3 months, unless the child is terminally ill. The need should be expected to continue for a further 6 months. The claim depends on the parents' assessment of how the illness or disability affects their child, which is the fundamental difference from the previous scheme when each child needed to be assessed by the doctor. The application form encourages the parents to submit supporting evidence from other relatives and involved professionals. If there is any doubt on receipt of the application, the Department of Social Security will arrange a consultation by their doctors.

It is important for all health professionals to be aware of the allowance and inform parents where applicable. Back-dated applications will not be accepted. The length of the form may be offputting and parents may need encouragement before applying.

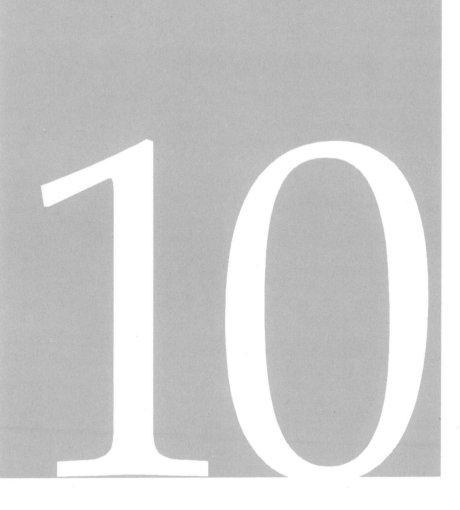

Epidemiology, statistics and audit

10

Audit

Q. You will be aware that audit has become increasingly used in medical practice. I wonder if you could tell me something about it.

Medical audit is essentially a process by which health professionals *assess, evaluate* and *improve* the care of patients in a systematic way. The 1989 Department of Health White Paper entitled *'Working for Patients'* was issued as part of the Government's NHS reforms and has led to the widespread mandatory use of audit within the profession. It defined medical audit as "the systematic critical analysis of the quality of medical care, including the procedures used for diagnosis and treatment, the use of resources and the resulting outcome and quality of life for the patient".

The audit process is best summarised by the audit cycle:

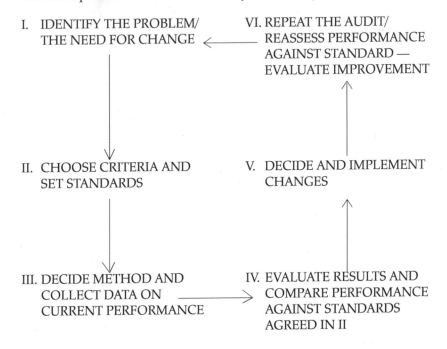

I. IDENTIFY THE PROBLEM/ THE NEED FOR CHANGE

VI. REPEAT THE AUDIT/ REASSESS PERFORMANCE AGAINST STANDARD — EVALUATE IMPROVEMENT

II. CHOOSE CRITERIA AND SET STANDARDS

V. DECIDE AND IMPLEMENT CHANGES

III. DECIDE METHOD AND COLLECT DATA ON CURRENT PERFORMANCE

IV. EVALUATE RESULTS AND COMPARE PERFORMANCE AGAINST STANDARDS AGREED IN II

Thus, audit is about self-improvement through standard setting and therefore implies change as well as measurement. Broadly speaking there are audits of *process* (investigating records to see how patients are being managed) and audits of *outcome* (investigating the results of management such as mortality and morbidity figures).

Audit may involve periodic review of recorded data such as case notes or analysis of outcome data such as perinatal mortality, discharges or post-mortem results or collection of previously unrecorded data such as patient satisfaction or assessment of patient education (e.g. diabetics). It also, of course, includes external audit.

An audit project which I carried out last year arose because I was concerned that children with acute asthma arriving in our A&E department were having to wait too long to receive their nebulised bronchodilators. After discussion with the paediatric and A&E consultants, I set our standards for maximum times and I then measured actual performance by analysing all affected children over 3 months. When I compared the two I was not surprised to find that we were only meeting our own standards in 56% of cases. With the help of the consultant paediatricians, I subsequently arranged a meeting with all staff concerned to discuss the reasons for this and decide how improvements could be made. A repeat of my audit 1 month later revealed that 92% of our acute asthmatics received their nebuliser within the maximum time.

Tip

■ It demonstrates both enthusiasm and wide experience if you can talk about a project that you have actually done.

Audit to reduce asthma admissions

Q. How could you use audit to reduce hospital admissions for acute asthma?

There is evidence of a large general increase in recent years in hospital inpatient rates for acute conditions. This appears to be related to a lowering of thresholds for admission rather than to a genuine increase in morbidity (Hill 1989). Audit should prove a useful tool for analysing patients in hospital and community practice for a variety of acute conditions, such as asthma, with the aim of finding methods for safely reducing admission rates.

First, I could use audit to assess procedures in the hospital admission room. I would record current patient details, including age, duration of illness, severity of attack as measured by objective criteria, treatment and admission rates. Outcome should also be established by way of duration of stay in hospital and peak flows over the ensuing days or weeks including after discharge. I would then repeat this after bringing about agreed alterations to the admission policy. One way to do this is to replace the admitting paediatrician with a more senior one.

A study was carried out along these lines in a Brighton hospital where the paediatrician responsible for admissions was changed from an SHO to an experienced registrar. Over 4 months, the rate of admission of patients with acute asthma fell form 84% to 66%. Diary symptom score cards filled in by parents indicated that children sent home without admission fared no worse than those who were first admitted (Connett et al 1993).

Similarly, I could use audit to assess various aspects of the general care of asthmatic children both in outpatient and in primary-care clinics. The correct use of national guidelines (in particular, adequate use of prophylactic measures, use of age-appropriate devices, inhaler technique, education of parents), the importance of temporarily increasing prophylaxis at the first signs of respiratory infection, compliance and attendance at clinics, could all be audited. I would repeat the audit after measures to improve these towards pre-determined standards had been implemented.

Thus, audit could be used both to improve the general standard of the long-term care of asthmatic children and admission policy, which will both result in a safe reduction in the number of acute admissions.

REFERENCES

Connett G J et al 1993 Audit strategies to reduce hospital admissions for acute asthma. Arch Dis Child 69: 202–205

Hill A M 1989 Trends in paediatric medical admissions. Br Med J 298: 1479–1482

Fundamental statistics

Q1. Why do we need statistics?

At its most basic, statistics is a measurement of chance. In most situations it is impossible to analyse a whole population (e.g. the age distribution of asthmatic children in Nottinghamshire). We therefore need to analyse a sample of this population and statistical analysis can indicate the degree of accuracy with which our sample reflects the population as a whole. This will be governed by the size of our sample and the nature of the distribution of our variable.

Statistics can also be used to assess the degree of difference between two groups of variables, e.g. the average morning peak flows of children during the weeks immediately before and after the addition of inhaled salmeterol to their therapy. The averages may appear higher after salmeterol but this apparent improvement may merely have been observed by chance. Statistics can be used to analyse the likelihood that this is the case and this is called statistical significance testing. Statistics is also used to ensure that results in medical research are comparable and generalised.

A doctor must have a basic knowledge of statistics if he/she intends to undertake any kind of research project or study. More importantly, most medical papers will employ statistical analysis and it is important that a medical reader is able to comprehend and critically evaluate the published results and conclusions.

Q2. How would you employ the services of a statistician?

I would discuss my proposed study with a statistician at the outset, once I had decided upon the broad objectives and I had some information about the populations concerned. He/she will be able to advise me on study design, data collection, randomisation, identification and minimisation of sources of error and bias. We will also decide the tests to be used before we start (thereby minimising the likelihood of encountering problems later on).

He/she will ensure that the study size is large enough to give a good chance of achieving statistical significance (i.e. advise on the power of the study). A statistician will also be able to advise on the design of questionnaires and the presentation of results and conclusions.

Q3. What is the difference between qualitative and quantitative data?

Data to which only a quality can be ascribed (and not an exact number) is said to be *qualitative*. This may be *nominal* (name only) such as male or female, dead or alive or blood group or *ranked* data (if they can be ordered in some way), such as severity of trauma.

Data to which a certain number can be ascribed is said to be *quantitative*. This may be *discrete* (if only certain discrete values are assumed), such as number of children, or *continuous* (assuming any value), such as plasma glucose.

Q4. What is a normal distribution?

The characteristics of the distribution of a variable are analysed by plotting frequency of the value on the vertical axis against the magnitude of the value on the horizontal axis. The variable is said to follow a *Normal* or Gaussian distribution if the plot is a smooth, characteristic bellshape which is symmetrical about the mean (i.e. the left- and right-hand halves are mirror images). In addition, the mean, median and mode values are all the same — the central value of the variable.

In practice, few if any variables in biological populations truly follow a Normal distribution, though we often make the assumption that they do.

Q5. What is a binomial distribution?

Data which can only take a 0 or 1 response, such as treatment success or failure, is said to follow a binomial distribution.

Q6. What are mean, median and mode values?

They are indicators of the central tendency of a distribution. The *mean* is the arithmetic average, i.e. sum of the values divided by number of values. The *mode* is the most commonly occurring value. The *median* is the middle value if all the values are placed in rank or ascending order.

Q7. What do you understand by the terms parametric and non-parametric tests?

If the variable under consideration approximately follows a normal distribution, than *parametric tests* of statistical significance are used. For example, the Student's *t*-distribution can be used in two ways. The paired *t*-test is used when paired or matched data are being examined such as in a matched case–control study or a cross-over trial (e.g. average peak flow before and after addition of new therapy). The unpaired *t*-test is used when the two groups in question are not connected. Examples of this situation are an unmatched case–control study or parallel group clinical trial.

If dealing with a non-normal distribution, then alternate tests must be employed and these are called distribution-free or *non-parametric tests*. In these situations, the unpaired *t*-test is replaced by the Wilcoxon test (also known as the Mann-Whitney U test) and the paired *t*-test is replaced by a Wilcoxon signed-rank sum test. These tests are tedious to calculate for large sample studies and computer packages are usually employed.

Non-parametric tests can always be used since no assumptions about the underlying population are made. However, if a near-Normal population can be assumed, it is better to use a parametric test as the calculated *p*-value will be smaller. Also, parametric tests are generally more flexible.

Q8. What is the null hypothesis?

The null hypothesis assumes that any apparent difference between two groups of variables has occurred by chance and that in reality, no difference exists and that the two groups are really from the same population. The *p*-value is a measure of the probability that the apparent difference has occurred by chance and different statistical tests can be applied to measure the *p*-value, depending on the nature of the data involved.

p-values range from 0.00 (0% likelihood that this has occurred by chance) to 1.00 (100% likelihood). We often arbitrarily employ a standard of 0.05 and if the *p*-value for the difference in two groups of variables (as calculated by an appropriately chosen statistical test) is less than this (i.e. there is a probability of <0.05 or <5% likelihood that this difference has occurred by chance), then we reject the null hypothesis. We therefore accept that there is a difference between the two groups (i.e. in the above example, that there is an improvement after the addition of salmeterol) and that the two groups of values do not come from the same population. This is statistical significance testing.

The statistical analysis does not really indicate the magnitude of any difference. If a low *p*-value has been obtained and the null hypothesis rejected, it merely reveals that a difference between two groups exists but not how large this is. It may in reality be smaller than, the same as or greater than the apparent differences as measured. Therefore, statistical significance does *not* mean biological or clinical significance. There may genuinely be an improvement in peak flow but this may be clinically so insignificant as not to justify introduction of a new therapy. Also, a *p*-value that looks highly impressive and appears to confirm a clinically significant and relevant difference does not tell all that needs to be known before modifying practice, i.e. nature of the study, how data were collected, randomisation, elimination of error and bias, etc!

Q9. What do you understand by variance and standard deviation?

The indicators of central tendency such as the mean give no idea about how widely dispersed the measured values of a variable are about the centre. The *variance* and *standard deviation* are both measures of scatter of data about the sample mean. The smaller they are, the less the natural scatter.

The variance is the average amount by which any individual value X differs from the mean ($\overline{X}$), and the standard deviation is the square root of the variance. The standard deviation can easily be used to calculate where values are distributed: 66% of values lie within the range $\overline{X} \pm 1$ SD; 95% of values lie within the range $\overline{X} \pm 2$ SD; 99% of values lie within the range $\overline{X} \pm 3$ SD.

Q10. What do you understand by the term standard error?

The standard error is a measure of the uncertainty of a simple statistical parameter. The commonest one is the standard error of the mean which is calculated by dividing the standard deviation by the square root of the number of values in the sample.

Q11. What are type I and type II errors?

Significance testing only indicates a balance of probabilities and therefore even conclusions drawn from statistical analysis can be wrong.

A *type I error* is basically a *false positive*. In other words, we have been lead to reject the null hypothesis and accept that there is a difference between two groups when in reality, one does not actually exist.

A *type II error* is basically a *false negative*. In other words, we have not rejected the null hypothesis when in reality, a genuine difference exists.

Q12. So, what do sensitivity and specificity mean?

These terms can be applied not only to statistical tests but also to clinical or biological ones, e.g. the Guthrie test. The probability that a test will correctly pick up a genuine positive result (i.e. when in reality a genuine difference between groups is present or disease is present) is the *sensitivity* of the test. The probability that a test will correctly indicate a negative result (i.e. when in reality no difference between groups or no disease is present) is the *specificity* of the test.

Q13. How does error differ from bias?

These two terms are quite separate and refer to different sources of inaccuracy in a study. *Bias* refers to systematic inaccuracy due to consistent over or under recording. This is usually due to recorder bias which may be completely subconscious. *Error* is any random source of inaccuracy at any stage of a study. For example, error in collecting variables merely leads to a less precise estimate of the value (in contrast with bias).

Error, because of its random nature, can usually be tackled by calculating it with appropriate statistical tests or simply by increasing the study size. Bias is a much more troublescme source of inaccuracy since its magnitude cannot readily be estimated. If discovered, removing bias is difficult and usually requires fundamental alteration of the study, notably the way data is collected. However, by its nature, it often goes unrecognised leading to erroneous conclusions.

Q14. What tests of statistical significance have you found most useful?

I have found the Student's t-test and the chi-squared test (χ^2 -test) most useful.

Q15. Tell me about the chi-squared test.

The chi-squared test is used to assess whether an observed distribution accords with that expected either on the basis of knowledge of the true population or on theoretical grounds. For example, if I were investigating a school with 356 boys and I found that of the 125 who lived on a housing-estate with marked social deprivation, 36 had asthma whereas of the 231 who lived elsewhere, only 44 had asthma, I could use the chi-square test to see if this is a significant difference. I would initially assume the null hypothesis that living on the housing-estate does not influence the likelihood of a child suffering from asthma and see if chi-square analysis disproves this.

It is important to remember that chi-squared tests may only be carried out on actual numbers of occurrences and not on percentages, proportions, means of observations or other derived statistics. Also, the chi-squared test does not require the assumption of a normal distribution.

Q16. Briefly tell me about t-tests.

t-tests are a commonly used statistical tool in various situations. (They were initially devised by WS Gosset in 1908 under the pseudonym 'Student' and they are sometimes referred to as 'Student's t-test'). They require the assumption of a Normal distribution but they have been specifically devised to handle data from small samples. t-tests assume a null hypothesis and are used to attempt to disprove this.

For example, they are often used when the means and standard deviations of two samples are known and the test is applied to see if there is a significant difference between the sample means (unpaired t-test). They may also be used for paired or matched samples (paired t-test).

Q17. What do you understand by the terms correlation and regression?

Correlation is the process of relating two quantitative variables (e.g. peak flow against height). I would do this by plotting the peak flow against the height for every individual studied. This produces a scatter diagram which will give a visual impression of any linear association between the two variables. Calculating the correlation coefficient would enable me mathematically to measure the strength of the linear association. This has a value between +1, which would indicate a perfect direct relationship and –1, which would indicate a perfect inverse relationship. A value at or around zero indicates no association.

Regression by contrast is a predictive process. Once a scatter diagram has been obtained for two such variables, the process of linear regression would allow me to draw the line of best fit. This would then enable me to predict the value of one of the variables for a given value of the other.

The two processes are complementary. Linear regression merely allows prediction of a variable from a given set of results but it does not indicate how likely that value is in reality. This is why we need the correlation coefficient since a high value (either + or –) suggests that there probably is an association and so the regression is credible.

Q18. What do you know about confidence intervals?

Confidence intervals define a range within which a given population parameter is likely to lie with a certain degree of certainty. The population parameter usually analysed is the mean and its confidence intervals are calculated from our sample mean and its standard error; in practice, a 95% confidence interval is often chosen.

Confidence intervals are based on the concept of predicting the results that we would obtain were we to repeat the study several times. Thus, if the study were to be repeated 100 times, of the 100 resulting confidence intervals, we would expect 95 of these to include the population mean.

Q19. What are the advantages of using confidence intervals rather than *p*-values?

Simple statements in reports such as $p < 0.05$ convey very little information about the results obtained from a study and create a rather artificial divide between 'significant' and 'non-significant'. 'Significance' relates purely to statistical significance which may not necessarily be ideal in the context of clinical studies.

Confidence intervals convey information about the magnitude of results obtained in a study together with an estimate of the precision with which a statistic estimates a population value. This is clearly very useful information for the reader and I have noticed that an increasing number of published articles report their findings using confidence intervals rather than tests of statistical significance.

British Paediatric Surveillance Unit

Q. Since 1986 there has been a consultant-led surveillance system for uncommon conditions in paediatrics. Can you tell me anything about it?

I believe you are referring to the British Paediatric Surveillance Unit (BPSU), as you say set up in 1986 to look at the incidence of the rarer and more unusual diseases affecting the paediatric population. Input is from the British Paediatric Association, the Public Health Laboratory Service, the Communicable Disease Surveillance Centre and the Department of Epidemiology.

Each month consultant paediatricians in the UK and Ireland receive a card listing the diseases under surveillance. They are requested to fill out the number of cases of the listed conditions seen in the previous month and to then return it to the BPSU office, even if the number of cases is zero.

Conditions that have been studied include:

1. HIV and AIDS
2. Reye's syndrome
3. Kawasaki's disease (discontinued in 1993)
4. Subacute sclerosing panencephalitis
5. Congenital rubella
6. Juvenile dermatomyositis
7. Androgen insensitivity syndrome
8. Invasive *Haemophilus influenzae* infection following Hib immunisation
9. Vitamin K deficiency bleeding

Researchers wishing to look at a rare condition can have the disease included on the monthly BPSU card. A part of the administrative cost must be paid for by the research team.

Facts and figures obtained can be very useful in planning future health care provisions, in understanding the natural history of conditions and then perhaps doing something to reduce the incidence. There is no better example of this than Reye's syndrome. Since Government recommendations that aspirin should not be prescribed to under 12 year olds there has been a significant reduction in the incidence of this condition.

Perinatal mortality

Q. What is perinatal mortality?

Perinatal mortality is the number of stillbirths plus the number of deaths at 0–6 days after live birth. It is said to be a reflection of the standard of maternity service care in a region or country. Perinatal mortality is therefore the responsibility of both obstetricians and paediatricians. There has been a steady reduction in the perinatal mortality rate in developed countries, which is due to a number of factors:

1. *Improved care of preterm infants* — there is a high correlation between perinatal mortality rate and the proportion of low birthweight infants. Advances in neonatal intensive care will therefore reduce the rate. However, a reduction in perinatal mortality may also mean an increase in morbidity of surviving low birthweight infants.

2. *Improved obstetric care* — with increased monitoring of the fetus during pregnancy, and particularly in labour, problems can be more easily anticipated. Labour may be accelerated, or a Caesarian section performed, and a paediatrician will be present at high-risk deliveries. There is a 6-fold increase in perinatal mortality following antepartum haemorrhage. There is also a greatly increased risk in multiple births, especially for the second infant.

3. *Reduction in congenital abnormalities* — many congenital abnormalities will be picked up by prenatal diagnostic procedures, such as ultrasound and amniocentesis or chorionic villus biopsy. With counselling, this may lead to termination of the pregnancy and therefore reduce early neonatal deaths.

4. *Parity* — there has been a trend for smaller families, which may have reduced perinatal mortality since high parity is strongly associated with increased risk of mortality.

5. *Maternal age* — there is a significantly lower risk of mortality if the mother is aged 20–29. There is a tendency for pregnancy to be confined to this more favourable age group.

There are some areas where the perinatal mortality rate remains higher than average. This may not be related to the obstetric/neonatal service, but to differences in the population. There is a close relationship between per capita income and perinatal mortality, with an increased risk for single mothers and those in social class V. However, the strongest relationship remains to low birthweight. It may be that some regions have a higher perinatal mortality rate due to a higher proportion of low birthweight babies, which again may be related to social circumstances. It may therefore be more appropriate to use birthweight-specific perinatal mortality rates when comparing regions.

There has previously been an anomaly in the calculation of the perinatal mortality rate, since live births before 28 weeks have been counted whereas those with no signs of life have not been counted as stillborn. This situation has now changed, as the definition of a stillbirth has been any infant born before 24 weeks. We should expect an increase in the perinatal mortality rate due to this change in definition.

Further reduction in perinatal mortality would be achieved by reducing the number of low birth weight infants born. However, the factors causing low birthweight and premature labour are still poorly understood. Research in this area should be beneficial. Increasing the availability of prenatal diagnosis and genetic counselling may also be helpful. Easy access to family planning services and improving neonatal care facilities is also important. A confidential enquiry into all perinatal deaths is being undertaken. This may be of interest in improving both obstetric and paediatric practice.

Definitions

$$\text{Perinatal mortality rate (per 1000 total births)} = \frac{\text{Still births (after 24 weeks)} + \text{early neonatal deaths (0–6 days)}}{\text{Total live and still births}}$$

Infant mortality rate = number of deaths in the first year per 1000 live births

Neonatal mortality rate = number of deaths in the first 28 days per 1000 live births

Screening

Q. If I am interested in screening the population for a particular condition, what is important for it to be worthwhile?

This question is best answered by dividing the answer into:

1. Particulars of the condition
2. Particulars of the screening test(s)

1. The disease/disorder in question must:
   — Have a natural history that is understood
   — Be important
   — Have a screening test that is available
   — Have an early asymptomatic stage
   — Have indications for treatment that are agreed
   — Have an acceptable and effective treatment
   — Be considered financially beneficial to screen for

2. The screening test being carried out must be:
   — Acceptable
   — Repeatable
   — Sensitive
   — Specific
   — Simple

Using examples of conditions that could potentially be screened for, it can be seen that it is not quite as straightforward as it may at first appear. Duchenne muscular dystrophy (DMD) is a very important condition, it being the commonest serious muscle disorder, with devasting effects on the patient and family. It has an incidence of ~1 in 5000, with about two-thirds having a positive family history. Screening for this condition has been possible since the late 1970s — blood taken on the Guthrie card at the end of the first week of life can be tested for creatine kinase. The test is simple, it is acceptable as the baby is having a heel prick anyway and it is repeatable. Specificity and sensitivity are a little more difficult to interpret as the condition has not been screened for, for a sufficient period of time as yet. The natural history of DMD is fully understood and there is an asymptomatic period. The only reason why it may not be worthwhile to screen for this condition, using the criteria above, is that there is, as yet, no effective and agreed treatment. Very little can be done to slow the progression of the disease, and it is invariably fatal, usually by the age of 20. Having said that, there are advantages to making the diagnosis in the newborn period. These include:

1. Enabling informed family planning
2. Avoidance of diagnostic delay and inappropriate investigation
3. Planning in advance care of the individual

Despite the fact that screening for DMD does not fit all the criteria, there is a very good argument for doing so. As the expectations and medical knowledge of the 'lay' population increase, the conditions diagnosable on the Guthrie card will inevitably grow and DMD quite probably will be one of them.

Medical studies

Q1. From your reading of the literature, what different forms do you think medical research can take?

The most powerful and convincing research takes the form of projects organised to analyse specific problems. These often have a statistical basis and may be observational (such as case–control or cohort studies) or interventional (such as clinical trials). Case reports and clinical observations do not strictly fall into the framework of statistical studies in medicine. However, despite their rather anecdotal nature, they are nevertheless a valuable source of medical information.

Q2. What are the main distinguishing features of medical studies?

The major classification of medical studies is into *longitudinal* or *cross-sectional* studies. Other distinguishing features are prospective or retrospective, randomised or non-randomised and interventional or observational.

Q3. What is the difference between longitudinal and cross-sectional studies?

A *longitudinal* study investigates processes over a defined period of time. *Cross-sectional* studies analyse a phenomenon fixed in time; in other words they describe a snap-shot picture.

Q4. Tell me about longitudinal studies.

Longitudinal studies may be *prospective* or *retrospective*. Clinical trials and cohort studies are examples of prospective studies.

In cohort studies, groups are studied forwards over a period of time and compared with respect to disease. The usual situation is to study two groups of people who have different exposure to a particular agent of interest (such as possible increased levels of radiation from nuclear plants), but are otherwise matched. The incidence of a particular disease (such as leukaemia) is compared in the two groups.

An example of a retrospective study would be a case-control study. This is where a group of people who have a specific disease (cases) are compared with those who do not and analysed to establish their past exposure to possible disease risk factors.

In other words case-control studies compare groups with respect to *exposure* whereas cohort studies compare groups with respect to *disease.*

Q5. What do you understand by the term clinical trial?

A clinical trial is defined as a prospective study to examine the relative efficacy of interventions such as treatments in *human* subjects. In most situations , this involves comparing standard treatment (the control group) with new therapy (the test group).

Q6. What are the factors that you would take into consideration when deciding upon and planning a clinical trial.

In deciding and planning a clinical trial, I would first and foremost look closely at my major objective and ensure that this was both clearly defined and clinically worthwhile. Once I was happy with this, I would look at any secondary objectives and ensure that these are also clearly stated.

Q7. What do you know about randomisation?

Randomisation is a procedure in which chance determines the assignment of a subject to the alternatives under investigation. The main reason for this is that randomisation produces study groups that are comparable in the unknown, hidden attributes as well as the known attributes which may influence the outcome in addition to the treatment itself. This therefore ensures that the probabilities obtained from statistical tests will be valid.

The process may take the form of simple randomisation such as tossing a coin to allocate patients or more complex techniques involving random number charts or computer programs. When the patient and his/her parents do not know which treatment is being used, this is called single-blind randomisation. When the doctor who is looking after the patient and assessing disease progress is unaware as well, this is called double-blind randomisation.

Q8. Tell me about cross-sectional studies.

Cross-sectional studies provide a 'snap-shot' view of a particular problem within a defined population. They provide no information about temporal relationships between the factors studied and usually involve the examination of a cross-section of a particular population at one point in time. Cross-sectional studies may be used to study associations between different diseases but they cannot determine which disease came first. Cross-sectional studies are also ideally suited to studying prevalence (which is the proportion of persons in a particular population who have a given disease). Broadly speaking, screening programmes are a form of cross-sectional study.

Although cross-sectional studies are less common than longitudinal studies in medical research, they are widely used in many areas of social analysis, including household surveys.

Paper criticism

Q. What factors go through your mind when you assess the quality of a paper in a journal and judge whether to alter your practice?

A knowledge of paper criticism is vital to a clinician for whom regular perusal of the journals is an integral part of continuing education. Even after a careful assessment of a paper, I have usually found it beneficial to 'sound out' my peers and consultants before actually changing my practice.

Broadly speaking, when I read a paper I ask myself three questions: were the objectives clearly set out and medically relevent?; was meticulous scientific method used throughout; and were the research objectives met?.

I would then consider the following points:

1. *General considerations:*   WHO CARES?.   SO WHAT ?.

    — Which journal is the paper in? Is it one of the 'major' ones?
    — Is it a refereed journal?
    — Who are the authors? Do they have a proven track record of meticulous research? – HOW BIG ARE THEIR HEADS?
    — How was the research sponsored? e.g. is there a pharmaceutical company (in which case there may be a questions mark over the degree of disinterest that the authors had in the study)?
    — Is there a well-written abstract (i.e. clearly setting out the objectives, study design, important results and main conclusions)?

2. *Objectives:*

    — Are the primary and secondary objectives clearly stated?
    — Are the objectives specific? I would ask myself "what are the authors actually trying to measures?"
    — Are these medically relevant?
    — Does the study build from existing theory? If so, has this been adequately validated (quality of referenced work)? and generally accepted?

3. *Study design:*

    — Sensible design?
    — Methods of recognising and minimising error and bias?
    — Duration of the study? Was it long enough reasonably to make the assessments and arrive at the conclusions in the study?
    — Completeness? How were 'missing subjects' or 'drop-outs' dealt with so as not to affect validity of sampling?

4. *Study sample:*

   — How obtained?
   — Representative?
   — Entry criteria and exclusions? Protocol?
   — How randomised, e.g. into control and study groups?
   — Is the control group acceptable?

5. *Measurements:*

   — Validity and reproducibility? How was the disease severity/treatment effectiveness assessed?
      — if 'human', what steps were taken to ensure accuracy and uniformity, e.g minimum number of 'assessing' doctors. Was there a protocol?
      — if using 'equipment', what steps were taken to ensure these were accurate and calibrated to have adequate sensitivity and specificity?
   — Blindness? single or double?
   — Quality control?

6. *Analysis:*

   — Was the analysis valid? e.g. if statistical analysis was used, was this done correctly (ideally with expert input)? Was the null hypothesis used and was the appropriate test applied?
   — Were any assumptions valid?
   — What do the statistical results really mean? Does this match-up with the way authors have interpreted the results?

7. *Conclusions and discussion:*

   — Are the conclusions reasonable based on the nature of the study itself?
   — Do the results support the conclusions?
   — Is there sufficient evidence to satisfy the criteria of a causal argument?
   — Did the study meet its objectives?

Tips

- This is not a question that you are likely to pass or fail on but the sort where demonstration of expertise is likely not only to bring valuable marks but also help in 'winning the examiners over'.

- We have listed several aspects of paper criticism. We would suggest that you outline the seven broad areas and then talk around some of the specific points.

Recent advances and controversial areas

11

Genetic research

Q. What does genetic research have to offer in the treatment of cystic fibrosis?

This question has a two-pronged answer:

1. Diagnosis of cystic fibrosis (CF)
2. Correction of the CF gene mutation

1. *Diagnosis of CF*

The majority of health authorities in the UK routinely screen for CF using Guthrie card blood taken on the 6th day of life. In the health authority I am working in, if the Guthrie card shows an elevated immunoreactive trypsin (IRT), then DNA analysis of the same blood sample is carried out, looking for the Δ F508 mutation (deletion of a phenylalanine residue at amino acid position 508 of the CFTR protein on the long arm of chromosome 7). Δ F508 is the gene mutation present in about 97% of patients with CF. Two-thirds of these are homozygous, the remaining one-third heterozygous, but in combination with another mutation of the same gene from the other parent. Those homozygous for Δ F508 have CF, but currently still undergo sweat test analysis to confirm the diagnosis. Those heterozygous for Δ F508 have a further IRT at 27 days — if still elevated, they have a sweat test.

Potential advantages from early diagnosis by neonatal screening include avoidance of unnecessary investigation and hospital admissions before the diagnosis is made, and genetic counselling for the parents. Disadvantages include the detection of carriers which could result in stigmatisation of that person. From another viewpoint, this would be considered an advantage, as if all carriers are detected now, in 16–18 years time, potential parents may not have children if they are known to be carriers.

2. *Correction of the CF gene mutation*

The CFTR (cystic fibrosis transmembrane conductance regulator) is a cAmp-regulated chloride channel. Dysfunction of the CFTR due to genetic mutations results in viscid mucus production at the luminal surface of secretory epithelium. If the abnormal CFTR gene can be mixed with a normal CFTR gene sequence, incorporated into cells, or cells can be produced with a normal CFTR gene sequence, then CF may be eradicated. More succinctly these methods can be described as somatic or germ-line therapies, respectively.

    a) *Somatic gene therapy*. This aims at treatment rather than prevention. By means of gene transfer systems, the normal CTFR gene sequence is incorporated into the relevant cells of the lungs, pancreas, sperm ducts and bilary tree, thereby producing normal chloride channel function. These gene transfer systems include viral vectors (adenovirus, HSV, vaccinia virus) and liposomes. Clinical trials are underway in the USA and in a few centres in the UK applying CFTR–cDNA/adenovirus recombinants to the nasal and bronchial epithelia.

Several issues arise to my mind from this:

— Unless stem cells are infected with the adenovirus then once the infected surface epithelial cells of the lungs die and are shed, repeated application of the virus vectors will be necessary.
— Only the respiratory problem of CF is being tackled by this method. Inhalation of the adenovirus will do nothing for pancreatic function or fertility (in males).
— What effect will integration of the virus into the host genome have on potential oncogenic processes in the infected cells.

b) *Germ-line therapy*. This would appear to have a redundant role in CF and it is hard to imagine it gaining prominence. For this to be feasible, the genetic material of the egg would need to be altered prior to fertilisation and implantation into the uterus. The gene mutation would require detection in the unfertilised egg, followed by incorporation of the normal CFTR gene sequence into the germ-line cells. Theoretically this would cure CF in offspring and also prevent passage of the gene mutation to further generations. Ethical reasoning must question tampering with germ-line cells, never mind the scientific feasibility of such endeavours.

REFERENCES

Coutlelle C et al 1993 Gene therapy for cystic fibrosis. Arch Dis Child 68: 437–443
Graham A, Geddes D M 1993 New developments in cystic fibrosis and their potential effects on its management. Curr Paed 3: 96–101

Techniques in genetic research

Q1. Name some techniques used in genetic research and molecular biology.

DNA hybridisation, which allows the use of gene probes, DNA fractionation or digestion and the polymerase chain reaction. The use of these techniques allows DNA to be mapped — normal and abnormal — in all chromosomes (the human genome project).

Q2. Tell me about DNA hybridisation.

This process utilises certain properties of DNA and RNA. First, the two strands of DNA can be dissociated and will reassociate (reanneal) specifically because of their complementary nucleic acid sequences. This can be done by heating and cooling. Secondly, if a small segment of DNA is manufactured which is complementary to a sequence found on one of the two strands (complementary DNA or cDNA), under suitable conditions it will search out and anneal only to that region. The region does not necessarily have to include the gene being investigated (for technical reasons this may be difficult) but merely lie close to it on the DNA strand (and move with it during cell division). If radioactive bases are attached to the synthesised cDNA, these specific regions can be identified and this is the principle of gene probes.

Q3. Tell me about DNA fractionation techniques and their uses.

DNA fractionation or digestion involves restriction endonucleases which are enzymes which occur naturally (mostly in bacteria) and which restrict themselves to only cleaving foreign DNA (i.e. not the bacteria's own). Specific endonucleases can be used which recognise only certain short sequences of DNA (restriction site). The DNA sequences between each restriction site are unique to each genome and these can be used to produce characteristic banding patterns on Southern blotting (restriction fragment length polymorphisms or RFLPs). This is therefore a powerful tool in gene research.

Polymerase chain reaction

Q. What do you know about PCR and its uses?

The polymerase chain reaction is an in vitro method of generating large amounts of a specific nucleic acid sequence and hence making subsequent analysis of that part of the genome much easier. Some prior knowledge of the sequence is required as the reaction is initiated by a pair of small synthetic nucleotide molecules (oligonucleotides) complementary to DNA sequences immediately adjacent to the area in question. The material containing the DNA is heated to cause dissociation of the two strands of the double helix and then cooled to allow the specific binding of the two oligonucleotides on either side of the region of interest. A DNA polymerase enzyme together with sufficient supply of nucleic acids is added to the 'broth' which then result in the generation of a copy of the DNA sequence between the two oligonucleotides. Repeated heating/cooling cycles thus lead to very large amounts of the specific region being reproduced which can then be analysed by techniques such as gel electrophoresis or DNA fragmentation.

The fundamental application of PCR is to establish the presence or absence of a specific DNA sequence and this allows the process to be used in the identification of pathogens (e.g. HIV, HBV, CMV, mycoplasma, etc.). PCR is an invaluable tool in the rapidly expanding field of prenatal and neonatal genetic diagnosis. The technique can be used to diagnose diseases such as cystic fibrosis and haemoglobinopathies and also to establish sex in the case of sex-linked disorders. PCR is also widely used in molecular biology and genetic research into various diseases involving gene mutations. Samples for PCR can range from urine, CSF, fine needle aspirates or any potentially infected material to chorionic villus biopsy, the Guthrie spot test or even pathological or post-mortem tissue.

Triplet repeats

Q1. What are triplet repeats?

DNA is made up of four nucleotides; adenine, guanine, thymine and cytosine. A sequence of these nucleotides (a codon) codes for an amino acid, e.g. CCT = glycine. In a number of genetic disorders, trinucleotides repeat more frequently than normal. Conditions identified so far include:

— Huntington's disease (chromosome 4)
— Fragile X (X chromosome)
— Dystrophia myotonica (chromosome 19)
— X-linked bulbospinal neuronopathy (X chromosome)

1. *Huntington's chorea.* The abnormality involves the expansion of the codon repeat of CAG from the normal 9–34, up to 100 at the distal short arm of chromosome 4. The length of the trinucleotide repeat and the age of disease onset are inversely correlated. Also, early onset is associated with paternal transmission because a larger number of CAG repeats are transmitted and also there is an association with expansion on transmission. This is the converse to transmission in dystrophia myotonica in which transmission from mother is associated with early onset and more severe disease. This also gives an explanation for anticipation (the tendency for autosomal dominant disease to be more severe in younger generations of a family).

2. *Dystrophia myotonica.* A CTG expansion of the long arm of chromosome 19. Transmission of the congenital form of dystrophia myotonica is almost exclusively from the mother, possibly due to an unidentified intrauterine factor or due to genomic imprinting effects. The normal repeat is 5–27, but in dystrophia myotonica it is 50–2000 or more.

3. *Fragile* X. A CGG expansion from the normal 6–54 to 52–200 in normal transmitting males and carrier females and up to 1000 in affected males. For every five affected males, there is another who inherits the gene without being affected (described as a normal transmitting male).

Q2. What about the genetics of Angelman's and Prader Willi syndromes?

Both conditions result from a deletion of chromosome 15 (15q 11–13), but have distinct clinical phenotypes. In *Angelman's* syndrome, typified by happy sociable affect, characteristic hand movements, epilepsy and very poor speech development, 75% occur de novo; parental chromosomes are normal, but the deletion of chromosome 15 in the child is always inherited from the mother. If the deletion occurs in the gene from the father, the child will have *Prader Willi* syndrome (obesity after the first year of life; hypotonia, hypogonadism, mental retardation). This is described as genomic imprinting, i.e. genetic information expressed differently depending on the parent of origin. In 2–3% of Angelman's, both chromosomes 15s are inherited from the father, no detectable deletions are found and this is described as uniparental disomy. 5% of cases will result from chromosomal rearrangements from the mother and a further 15% have no detectable abnormality of genetic material. In Prader Willi, about 50% of affected cases show the deletion of chromosome 15 transmitted from the father on high solution banding techniques. 5% have duplications or translocations and the remainder have normal karyotypes.

REFERENCES

Clayton-Smith J 1992 Angelman's syndrome. Arch Dis Child 67: 889–891
Donaldson M D C et al 1994 The Prader Willi syndrome. Arch Dis Child 70: 58–63
Harding A E 1993 The gene for Huntington's disease. Br Med J 307: 396–397
Harley H G et al 1992 Unstable DNA sequences in myotonic dystrophy. Lancet 339: 1125–1128
Reardon W et al 1993 The natural history of myotonic dystrophy: mortality and long term clinical aspects. Arch Dis Child 68: 177–181

Free radicals

Q. What do you know about free radicals?

Free radicals are highly reactive chemical species which possess an unpaired electron. They represent fragments of molecules or atoms and may be negatively or positively charged or neutral. They are denoted chemically by convention with a heavy dot next to the symbol for the species. Free radicals arise in the body either deliberately during phagocytosis or accidentally during metabolic reactions.

They are usually produced in cells by electron transfer reactions except in the unusual circumstances under the influence of ionising radiation. The most important free radicals are oxygen free radicals, such as the superoxide radical O_2^- and the hydroxyl radical $OH^\bullet$. Other examples are carbon-centred and sulphur-containing free radicals.

Free radicals do have an important physiological role in inflammation and phagocytosis where their generation from neutrophils is linked to the action of NADPH oxidase. Abnormal NADPH oxidase activity leads to chronic granulomatous disease and these individuals have defective bacterial defences and are at risk of, for example, overwhelming staphylococcal infection.

Free radicals are usually, however, unwanted as they are potentially damaging to the body and their involvement in a variety of disease states is becoming increasingly recognised. Oxidation is the major damaging effect of free radicals and various protective mechanisms exist against them which are therefore termed antioxidant defences. Some of these are preventive such as efficient electron transfer systems. Others are scavenging or interceptive and these include vitamin E (tocopherol), vitamin C (ascorbic acid) and superoxide dismutase (the only enzyme whose substrate is free radicals).

There is increasing evidence for a pathogenic role of free radicals in such diverse diseases as carcinogenesis, shock-related tissue injury, α_1-antitrypsin-deficiency-mediated lung disease, muscular dystrophy and inflammatory joint disease.

Free radicals are thought to have a role in various neonatal diseases. They are proposed to be at least partly responsible for the pathogenesis of retinopathy of prematurity. However, trials investigating the use of antioxidants in prevention have shown that vitamin E is unfortunately 'not a panacea' (Phelps et al 1987).

Similar pathogenetic mechanisms have been proposed for free radicals in intraventricular haemorrhage (IVH) and in hypoxic ischaemic encephalopathy (HIE). Data relating to the prevention of IVH in premature infants with antioxidants is generally conflicting although some studies have shown promising results with a reduction in all grades of damage (Chiswick et al 1983, Sinha et al 1987).

Free radicals appear to be generated during hypoxic ischaemic encephalopathy and thus can produce additional damage. They can attack fatty acid components of cell membranes and inhibitors or scavengers of free radicals may have a role in the treatment of this condition (Vaccucci 1990, Volpe 1989).

Thus, research into the role of free radicals in various diseases and the potential benefits of protecting the body against them promises to be exciting. However, the facts that free radicals are usually produced close to their site of potential damage and they are very short-lived in body tissues means that they are difficult moieties to investigate.

REFERENCES

Chiswick M L et al 1983 Protective effect of vitamin C in intraventricular haemorrhage in premature babies. Br Med J 287: 81–84

Phelps D L et al 1987 Tocopherol efficacy and safety for prevention of retinopathy of prematurity: a randomised double-masked trial. Pediatrics 79: 489–500

Sinha S et al 1987 Vitamin C supplementation reduces the frequency of periventricular haemorrhage in very preterm babies. Lancet 1: 466–470

Vaccucci R C 1990 Current and potentially new management strategies for perinatal hypoxic ischaemic encephalopathy. Pediatrics 85: 961–968

Volpe J J 1989 Intraventricular haemorrhage and brain injury in the premature infant; neuropathology and pathogenesis. Clin Perinat 16: 361–386

Steroids in meningitis

Q1. Do you think we should be using dexamethasone routinely in bacterial meningitis?

Bacterial meningitis is still a common problem in Britain, with an overall mortality of 10%. It also causes morbidity due to sensorineural deafness, epilepsy and other neurological sequelae. Progress is being made with respect to prevention of meningitis by active immunisation against causative organisms, e.g. *Haemophilus influenzae* and tuberculosis. However, despite powerful antibiotic regimens, there has been little improvement in morbidity in recent years.

It is thought that much of the cerebral damage may be caused by activation of the host inflammatory pathways in response to the bacteria, rather than the organism itself. Inflammation occurs when the endotoxin produced by the bacteria induces the inflammatory cascade. Synthesis and release of the cytokines can be blocked in vitro by the addition of dexamethasone to cultured cells. Animal studies show that the inflammatory response is dampened when dexamethasone is given before, but not after, antibiotics.

Several clinical studies have suggested that neurological sequelae are reduced in children treated with dexamethasone prior to antibiotics, but the results are not statistically significant. When the analysis was restricted to cases of meningitis caused by *Haemophilus influenzae*, there was a significant reduction in hearing loss. The use of dexamethasone in meningococcal meningitis, which is becoming the more common cause of meningitis in children due to the introduction of an immunisation schedule for haemophilus, is less clear. Mortality in meningococcal disease remains high and this difference may be related to the accompanying septicaemia which leads to septic shock. The use of steroids in other types of septic shock may be harmful, so more evidence is required before recommending the use of dexamethasone in meningococcal disease. There is, as yet, little evidence for the use of steroids in other types of meningitis, e.g. pneumococcal or neonatal meningitis, due to the low numbers involved.

Measures of inflammation, such as temperature, cerebrospinal glucose and protein and neutrophil count, have been shown to improve more rapidly in children treated with steroids, so a reduction in morbidity would be expected. The addition of steroids to treatment regimens has not been shown to delay the rate of cerebrospinal fluid sterilisation. The side-effects of using high dose intravenous dexamethasone seem to be relatively few in the short courses used. However, gastrointestinal bleeding has occurred.

In conclusion, the use of dexamethasone as adjunctive therapy in bacterial meningitis may reduce morbidity, but larger studies are required to prove whether this is the case. A prolonged follow-up period will be needed fully to assess the usefulness of steroids. I have not worked in a unit where dexamethasone is used routinely.

Q2. If the decision is made to use dexamethasone, how would you administer it?

To benefit from the full anti-inflammatory effect of dexamethasone, it needs to be given intravenously at least 10 minutes prior to giving antibiotics. The dose is then repeated 6–12 hourly over a period of at least 2 days. It is important not to delay treatment of meningitis in the sick child and it may be considered inappropriate to delay giving antibiotics in the child with shock who appears clinically to have meningococcal disease.

Restriction fragment length polymorphism

Q. What is your understanding of restriction fragment length polymorphism?

Bacteria contain restriction enzymes which prevent incorporation of foreign DNA into host DNA. These enzymes recognise and cleave at a unique recognition site which is specific for a DNA sequence, e.g. GAATTC for EcoRI (*Escherichia coli*), which causes cleavage between guanine and cytosine of the DNA sequence. Many hundreds of thousands or even millions of fragments may be produced, all of variable length, but with a common base sequence at one or both ends. Electrophoresis of the fragmented DNA soup will result in separation of the different molecularly charged pieces. Identical DNA would produce an identical electrophoretic strip, but if mutations are present in the gene sequence, fragmentation will produce pieces of genetic material of different lengths again and a different electrophoretic picture. This difference in fragmentation is called a restriction fragment length polymorphism (RFLP).

The technique of RFLP is useful in looking at the inheritance of a condition within a family, once the family is identified. For example, if a boy is found to have Wiskott-Aldrich syndrome (thrombocytopaenia, eczema and T-cell deficiency), then performing RFLP on other family members can identify carriers and those that may become affected, should there be a long latent, asymptomatic period. Antenatal diagnosis can be undertaken if fetal blood sampling is performed. To its disadvantage, RFLP is not always able to detect abnormality, especially if cleavage of the DNA takes place some distance from the gene defect/mutation. The relatively recent advance of RFLP as a genetic test is probably now outdated as the techniques of molecular genetics advance at such an incredible pace.

Cochlear implants

Q. Paediatric cochlear implantation is being increasingly developed and used by ENT surgeons. Tell me about this technique.

A cochlear implant is essentially a sophisticated hearing aid which bypasses the inner-ear hair cell system and stimulates the ganglion cells of the VIIIth cranial nerve directly. It is indicated as a management option for profound sensorineural hearing loss which is a common problem with a prevalence in children in the UK between 1 and 2 per 1000. In practice, the commonest cause of acquired loss is meningitis. In addition, it is now increasingly being used to treat prelinguistic deafness such as children with congenital deafness.

It is widely accepted that the technique should only be employed where conventional amplification and rehabilitation methods have failed. However, there is controversy over the level of hearing loss; total loss of hearing with aided responses at thresholds >60 dB across the frequency range from 500 Hz–4 kHz is used in the Nottingham programme.

The surgical technique consists of implanting an electrode array directly into the cochlear with a receiver package lying in the post-aural region; sometimes an extracochlear electrode is used. Speech signals are transmitted to the receiver package by electromagnetic induction from a small coil held over the receiver by a magnet. Sound is received and modified through a small body-worn microphone/speech-processor unit before being transmitted to the receiver.

The benefits of cochlear implantation are potentially far-reaching. The primary benefits are detection of sound and speech at comfortable levels and enhanced lip-reading skills. Secondary benefits are improved voice and speech quality. Gibbin (1992) has outlined likely tertiary benefits such as improved educational and intellectual development and employment prospects.

However, it is important to bear in mind that cochlear implantation does not start and end with the surgical procedure. A team approach is essential involving a surgeon, speech therapist, teacher of the deaf, audiologist, medical physicist and, in particular, the child's parents. The feelings and expectations of parents need to be carefully assessed and careful counselling is critical, especially in relation to the long-term rehabilitation programme and the predicted extent of benefits. It must be remembered that an implant does not restore normal hearing. Older recipients state that there is great improvement in their quality of life but still describe the resulting sound as distorted.

REFERENCE

Gibbin K P 1992 Paediatric cochlear implantation. Arch Dis Child 67: 669–674

Viva topic survey

Neonatology

1. What factors would you take into consideration when designing a neonatal unit?
2. How would you investigate portal hypertension in neonates?
3. Innovations in infant feeding–use of long-chain fatty acids.
4. How would you investigate and manage a 36 week premature infant with respiratory distress?
5. What are you looking for when examining the anterior fontanelle in a newborn baby check?

Cardiology and respiratory medicine

1. Bronchiolitis — principles of management.
2. Investigation and management of hypertension in a 10 year old.
3. Outpatient management of asthma.

Endocrinology, growth and renal medicine

1. Management of congenital hypothyroidism.
2. Therapeutic uses of growth hormone.
3. How would you know if your diabetic clinic was effective (hint...Audit !).

Clinical pharmacology and therapeutics

1. When would you use penicillin in paediatrics?
2. Steroid use in the treatment of meningitis.

Neurology, psychiatry, community paediatrics and ethics

1. Changing dietary habit in toddlers.
2. Management of recurrent febrile convulsions.
3. Investigation of infantile spasms.
4. Management of glue ear.
5. Health of the Nation — implications.
6. The Patient's Charter — implications.

7. Parent-held records — pros and cons.
8. Management of strabismus.
9. The Fragile X syndrome.
10. Assessment of development problems in infancy.

Epidemiology, statistics and audit

1. Odds ratios.
2. Mortality figures.

Clinical governance

- A framework through which the NHS org. are accountable for continuously improving the quality of service & safeguarding high Stds of care by creating an environment in which excellence in clinical care will flourish

Glossary

As far as possible, you should avoid abbreviations in the viva as this tends to make you sound flippant. However, we have used some of the commoner ones to reduce the volume of the text.

ADH	Antidiuretic hormone
AIDS	Acquired immunodeficiency syndrome
ASD	Atrial septal defect
BP	Blood pressure
BPA	British Paediatric Association
CAH	Congenital adrenal hyperplasia
CHD	Congenital heart disease
CMV	Cytomegalovirus
CT	Computerised tomography (scan)
CXR	Chest X-ray
DHCC	Dihydroxycholecalciferol
DIC	Disseminated intravascular coagulation
DKA	Diabetic ketoacidosis
DNA	Deoxyribonucleic acid
EBV	Epstein-Barr virus
ECG	Electrocardiogram
ECMO	Extracorporeal membranous oxygenation
EEG	Electroencephalogram
ENT	Ear, nose and throat
ESR	Erythrocyte sedimentation rate
FBC	Full blood count
GFR	Glomerular filtration rate
GI	Gastrointestinal
Hb	Haemoglobin
HIE	Hypoxic ischaemic encephalopathy
HIV	Human immunodeficiency virus
ICP	Intracranial pressure
INR	International normalised ratio (for prothrombin time)
IQ	Intelligence quotient
ITU	Intensive therapy unit
IVH	Intraventricular haemorrhage
JVP	Jugular venous pulse
LFT	Liver function tests
NAI	Non-accidental injury
NG	Nasogastric
PCR	Polymerase chain reaction

PDA	Patent ductus arteriosus
PE	Pulmonary embolus
PEFR	Peak expiratory flow rate
PICU	Paediatric intensive care unit
PKU	Phenylketonuria
PR	Per-rectal examination
PTH	Parathyroid hormone
PUO	Pyrexia of unknown origin
RDS	Respiratory distress syndrome
SBR	Serum bilirubin
SHO	Senior house officer
SIADH	Syndrome of inappropriate ADH secretion
SIDS	Sudden infant death syndrome
SLE	Systemic lupus erythematosus
SVT	Supraventricular tachycardia
U&E	Urea and electrolytes
UTI	Urinary tract infection
VSD	Ventricular septal defect

Index